About the Author

For over 20 years, Dr Marilyn Glenville has practised nutrition in the UK and USA. She specialises in the natural approach to female hormone problems   ıns clinics in London and Kent. She is one of the UK's leading ex   in nutritional health for women.

As a respected authority on women's healthcare, Dr Glenville gives regular talks on radio and has often appeared on television and in the press. She frequently advises health professionals and lectures at academic conferences held at the Medical Society and the Royal College of Physicians. She obtained her doctorate from Cambridge University and is a Fellow of the Royal Society of Medicine and a member of the Nutrition Society.
Dr Glenville has been officially appointed by the Foods Standards Agency to be an observer on the Expert Group on the safety of Vitamins and Minerals. She is also a steering group member of the Forum on Food and Health at the Royal Society of Medicine.

Dr Glenville's previous books include the bestselling *Natural Solutions to Infertility, Nutritional Health Handbook* (both Piatkus), *Natural Alternatives to HRT* and *Natural Alternatives to Dieting*.

OTHER BOOKS BY THIS AUTHOR:

Nutritional Health Handbook for Women (Piatkus, 2001)
Natural Solutions to Infertility (Piatkus, 2000))
Natural Alternatives to HRT (Kyle Cathie, 1999)
Natural Alternatives to HRT Cookbook (Kyle Cathie, 1999)
Natural Alternatives to Dieting (Kyle Cathie, 1999)
Natural Choices for Menopause (St Martin's Press, 1999)

Natural Solutions to PMS

Marilyn Glenville PhD

PIATKUS

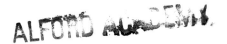

Visit the Piatkus website!

Piatkus publishes a wide range of exciting fiction and non-fiction, including books on health, mind body & spirit, sex, self-help, cookery, biography and the paranormal. If you want to:

- read descriptions of our popular titles
- buy our books over the Internet
- take advantage of our special offers
- enter our monthly competition
- learn more about your favourite Piatkus authors

visit our website at:
www.piatkus.co.uk

To Janet and Terry – you are close to my heart

Contents

Acknowledgements

My thanks go to Karen Sullivan for her persistence in asking me questions and helping to make the book so clear. I would also like to thank Alice Davis, Sandra Rigby and Judy, Gill and Philip at Piatkus for their continued interest and support.

Special thanks go to my practice staff, including Linda McVan, my wonderful practice manager and to Brenda, Mel, Nicola and Jacqui. My love goes to my family, my husband Kriss and my children Matthew, Leonard and Chantell who are always encouraging and who could probably do well in a quiz where their specialist subject was 'female hormone problems'!

My gratitude goes to my patients who over the years have opened up their hearts and thoughts to me, and their honesty has been really appreciated. What has been so revealing is their marvellous sense of humour and willingness to try a different approach.

PART ONE

THE PMS PUZZLE

Introduction

It isn't just your imagination – or the fact that it's Monday morning. Getting out of bed is such an effort and at breakfast you snap at your children or partner. As you head out of the door, bloated and grumpy, you don't know how you will get through the day and by the middle of the afternoon you have eaten a whole packet of biscuits and a couple of chocolate bars.

Sound familiar? If you've been feeling something like this around the middle of your monthly cycles, you could have premenstrual syndrome – and you're not alone. The condition affects up to 90 per cent of women before they reach the menopause. PMS, it has to be said, has had a terrible press, and women who suffer from it have sometimes been portrayed as red-eyed monsters on the rampage. For the vast majority of sufferers, however, PMS is much less dramatic, while still remaining a definite problem in their lives.

The term 'PMS' describes any symptoms that happen between ovulation and the start of the period. And there are over 150 of them, from food cravings, breast tenderness, headaches and irritability to mood swings and crying spells. They can come in all sorts of combinations, and range from mildly annoying to very severe.

You may decide you can just live with them. But if PMS is preventing you from working and playing as freely as you'd like, you'll need to take a harder look at what you can do about it. That's where this book comes in.

In Part One we'll be looking at causes, symptoms, diagnoses and conventional treatments for PMS. But first, let's glance at the PMS puzzle – the confusions and ambiguities surrounding a condition that for many of us remains all too real.

Not just all in the mind

Because PMS involves so many symptoms – which seem to increase yearly – it has been difficult to pin down. And there are other problems. The symptoms begin in the days leading up to a period, and disappear when a period begins. And yet when doctors examined one group made up of women with PMS and one group without, and measured hormone levels in the second half of their cycles, they found no difference in the two groups' hormone profiles.

What's more, despite the fact that PMS was officially recognised seventy years ago, there is still no clear understanding of what causes it. Even more confusing is the fact that every treatment (and, to date, there are more than eighty on offer) used for the condition seems to have a beneficial effect. And that the placebos, or dummy treatments, given in trials often perform better than the active treatment itself – sometimes with a 94 per cent success rate,[1] although the results are often short-lived.

This dilemma has clouded the research and treatment of the condition over the years. In 1993, the debate over PMS became so heated that some experts even suggested that it wasn't a medical condition at all, but merely a psychological problem – 'all in the mind'. It was proposed that women everywhere were claiming they had PMS when they were really just in a bad mood. These researchers argued that if women believe they have the condition, they become conditioned to blame mood swings, depression and aggression on it. So it becomes a self-fulfilling prophecy.

Were they wrong? Certainly, if some 94 per cent of women felt that their PMS symptoms were improved by taking nothing more than a sugar pill, there must be a psychological element to the condition. But it's not the whole story.

Whatever the case, women are in a no-win situation. If PMS *does* exist, we are forced to acknowledge that women will feel, behave and cope differently depending on the day of the month. Given that women have been fighting long and hard to prove that our different physiology is no barrier to achievement, it's difficult to argue that we will be as effective as men if we have a monthly hurdle to meet. On the other hand, if PMS does not exist, then we have been making excuses, and blaming erratic behaviour on hormones, without just cause. So where does this leave us?

I believe that PMS is a very real problem, and I'm not alone. Along with the studies that estimate it affects 70 to 90 per cent of women during their reproductive years[2] are others indicating that some 30 to 40 per cent of women have physical and psychological symptoms severe enough to inter-fere with their lives.

In fact, as many of us have heard, some women with PMS can undergo Jekyll and Hyde transformations so extreme that they have been used as mitigation in murder trials. A number of women have even been spared jail sentences on condition that they were given treatment. But these cases are thankfully few, and the worst consequences most women with PMS suffer are missed days of work, or a bad argument with a loved one.

A growing problem?

There are certainly many more reported cases of PMS than there were just a few years ago. This might be because we are more aware of the condition, so it gets a speedier diagnosis. On the whole, however, I would say that PMS is more common than it was a few generations ago because women are having more menstrual cycles.

Decades ago, when bigger families were the norm, women were preg-nant for many of their childbearing years, and then breastfed each child for many months. Because breastfeeding stops menstruation, some women used it as a form of contraception for some time after the birth of each child. Then these women would become pregnant again. So they hardly had a chance of experiencing premenstrual symptoms, because they simply weren't having as many cycles.

In the West these days, of course, families are a lot smaller and fewer women are caught up in this strenuous cycle of pregnancies. Many more women are also pursuing careers, often well into their thirties, and thus put having children on the back burner. These women could have had up to twenty years of periods between the ages of fifteen and about thirty-five, with no break. So they're much more likely to become aware of monthly symptoms. Added to this, girls now tend to start having periods earlier than they did in previous generations – some even at the tender age of eight.

This, too, will increase the number of menstrual cycles a woman will have throughout her life.

To look at it another way, the average women has periods for between thirty-five and forty years of her life, amounting to seven years of menstruation. So if a woman has PMS before each of these periods, she'll have experienced seven years of misery. PMS, in other words, is difficult to miss.

Why me?

What causes PMS? The real answer is that nobody knows. The cure would be obvious if we knew the cause, but our knowledge remains inconclusive.

Most researchers have been seeking a premenstrual 'holy grail' – a single mechanism that causes PMS. But as we've seen, this seventy-year crusade has failed, even though a number of treatments have been found to alleviate certain symptoms of PMS in placebo-controlled trials. And a vast range of treatments have been tested – from progesterone, oestrogen and vitamin E to reflexology, light therapy and evening primrose oil. The fact that such a varied range of treatments work for particular symptoms seems to indicate that the 'holy grail' approach is futile. Perhaps it's time to accept the fact that there is no single cause or cure. And this would end the situation where women are shuttled around between gynaecologist, endocrinologist and psychiatrist just to get a diagnosis.

What emerges from all this is the fact that women are not simply a collection of 'bits' that can be analysed and altered. Every system in the human body is interrelated, and by treating only one aspect – hormones, for example, or emotional health – we will never reach the crux of the problems associated with PMS. It's necessary to look at the whole woman – mind and body – for treatment to be successful. Most importantly, it has to be accepted that every woman is unique, and that the cause of any condition, including PMS, is unique to her.

This holistic approach to PMS has been highly successful, so much so that even the traditionalists have been forced to acknowledge the fact. As a specialist writing in the *Journal of Psychosomatic Obstetrics and Gynaecology* has said, 'Human behaviour cannot be understood within a single . . . frame of reference. Unravelling the [development] of PMS requires a multi-disciplinary approach.'[3]

This book shows how wonderfully effective the holistic approach is at untangling and treating the complex and interwoven symptoms of PMS.

_____

CHAPTER 1

What Is PMS?

If PMS is often seen as a slippery customer, difficult to diagnose and treat, some of its mystery could be rooted in how women were viewed in ancient times. To many early peoples, there was something awe-provoking in menstruation itself – the ability of women to bleed regularly without dying. In these cultures, women's blood was viewed as a confirmation of the miracle of life. Women were believed to be so powerful that they were required to remove themselves from their communities when they were menstruating. Some cultures also recognised the close connection between the cycle of the moon and a woman's monthly cycle, deepening its mythological meaning.

PMS came to light much later, as we'll see in the brief history that follows. Then we'll be looking at how we define the condition today.

Putting a name to it

PMS isn't a new phenomenon. As early as the 4th century BC, Hippocratic physicians were noting women's physical and psychological symptoms during their cycle.[1] In Victorian times the psychiatrist Sir Henry Maudsley described the condition, writing, 'The monthly activity of the ovaries which marks the advent of puberty in women has a notable effect on the mind and body: wherefore it may become an important cause of mental and physical derangement.'[2] But it wasn't until 1931 that an American neurologist, Robert Frank, first introduced the idea of an actual health condition relating to the female cycle. Presenting his theories to the New York Academy of Medicine, Frank suggested that this condition, which he called premenstrual tension (PMT), was caused by faulty function in the ovaries.[3] In the same year, a psychoanalyst also acknowledged the problem, but suggested that it was the result of suppressed sexual desire and power.[4]

The name 'PMT' stuck for a long time, even though tension was merely part of the story. But during the 1930s and 1940s, only the emotional symptoms associated with the menstrual cycle, such as irritability or anxiety, were noted.

A breakthrough came in 1953, when the premenstrual pioneer Dr Katharina Dalton, along with Dr Raymond Greene, published the first significant piece to describe PMS, in the *British Medical Journal*.[5] Dalton suggested that the condition's name be changed to 'premenstrual syndrome' or PMS, to reflect the fact that it wasn't a single health condition, but a syndrome, or group of symptoms characterising a condition, of which tension was only one. Today both names are used interchangeably, but PMS is by far the more accurate.

So much for the condition's bumpy history. Now it's time to take a closer look at the cluster of symptoms that make up PMS.

Pinning down the symptoms

'What's the difference between a woman with PMS and a terrorist? You can negotiate with a terrorist.'

PMS jokes are legion, but for many women, the symptoms are no laughing matter. Sometimes, as we'll see later, they are so serious that they disrupt family life, put children's lives in danger, and even cause marriages to break up. It's estimated that 70 to 90 per cent of women are affected every month by premenstrual symptoms – and that between 30 and 40 per cent of women suffer symptoms debilitating enough to interfere with their daily lives.[6]

The 150 symptoms coming under the PMS umbrella can be broken down into two groups – the physical and the psychological.

Physical symptoms

- Sugar and food cravings
- Bloating
- Water retention
- Breast tenderness and swelling
- Dizziness

- Tiredness
- Acne
- Headaches/migraines
- Weight gain
- Clumsiness
- Lack of co-ordination
- Aches and pains
- Dizziness or vertigo
- Fainting
- Changes in sex drive
- Tremors
- Excessive thirst
- Palpitations
- Changes in sleep patterns, such as insomnia, restlessness and heavy or prolonged sleeping
- Nausea
- Vomiting
- Lower back pain
- Cramps
- Bowel changes, including constipation or diarrhoea
- Runny nose
- Sore throat
- Vaginal discharge or thrush
- Accident-prone behaviour
- Alcohol intolerance
- Eye problems, such as styes and conjunctivitis
- Herpes (oral or genital)
- Piles (haemorrhoids)
- Hives (itchy skin)
- Light or noise intolerance
- Restlessness or jitteriness

Emotional/psychological symptoms

- Mood swings
- Irritability
- Anxiety
- Tension

- Anger
- Aggression
- Depression
- Crying spells
- Forgetfulness
- Suicidal tendencies
- Inability to cope
- Poor concentration
- Panic attacks
- Confusion
- Lethargy
- Agoraphobia (fear of open or public spaces)
- Feelings of insecurity
- Feelings of low self-worth
- Loss of self-esteem
- Indecisiveness
- Paranoia
- Fearfulness
- Illogical thinking
- Irrational thoughts
- Hallucinations
- Delusions
- Jealousy
- Feelings of guilt
- Poor judgement
- Loneliness

If this is starting to look too negative, there is another side to the coin. Some women have commented on positive changes in the lead-up to menstruation, such as their feeling energetic and in control, and managing satisfying bouts of cleaning and tidying up. Artists and writers often comment that for them, it is a very creative time of the month when ideas are flowing freely. They may even feel that they are in a different state of consciousness, where their perceptions are heightened.

How long do the symptoms last? PMS can vary in duration with women's cycles. A women with a cycle every thirty-five days could be ovulating on day 18 and have seventeen days' worth of premenstrual symptoms. Meanwhile, a woman with a twenty-one-day cycle, who ovulates on day 14, may suffer only seven days of PMS – but she will experience the symptoms more frequently because she will only just have got rid of them when the whole cycle begins again. Most women find that the symptoms only lift as their periods get into full flow. It's as if the release of the blood provides the release of the symptoms. And, interestingly, women who 'spot' before their periods do not experience a relief of symptoms until their periods start properly.

In any case, for all women with PMS, the symptoms do disappear completely for part of the month. This means that for one week or so every month, women with PMS feel 'normal' and happy, can cope with life, and have the energy to do the things they want to do.

The search for a system

A syndrome that sports 150 symptoms and varies from woman to woman can be a doctor's nightmare. So back in the early 1980s, Dr Guy Abraham tried to make classifying PMS easier with a system of four categories for the different types of symptoms. He suggested that each category is caused by its own hormonal imbalance.[7] Abraham's system is described below.

Type A: Anxiety

Abraham claimed this category is very common in up to 80 per cent of all women with PMS, and includes symptoms such as mood swings, irritability, anxiety and tension.

Suggested cause: An imbalance of oestrogen and progesterone, with the oestrogen levels being too high and those of progesterone too low.

Type C: Cravings

This group of symptoms, Abraham said, includes cravings for sweets, an increased appetite, fatigue and headaches. Up to 60 per cent of women with PMS can experience them.

Suggested cause: Problems with glucose tolerance. Glucose tolerance tests are abnormal in the five to seven days before menstruation, but normal the rest of the month.

Type H: Hyperhydration

Type H includes symptoms such as water retention, breast tenderness and swelling, abdominal bloating and weight gain. Up to 40 per cent of women with PMS can experience these changes.

Suggested cause: An excess of aldosterone, a hormone released by the adrenal glands that act on the kidneys to regulate water balance.

Type D: Depression

Depression is the prevalent symptom in this group, according to Abraham, but it also includes other related symptoms, including confusion, forgetfulness, clumsiness, feeling withdrawn, lack of co-ordination, paranoia and crying spells. Only 5 per cent of women suffering from PMS experience these symptoms, but it can be the most serious of the four groups if there are suicidal tendencies.

Suggested cause: Too little oestrogen and too much progesterone.

There are, however, a number of difficulties with Abraham's simple classification. For one, it is physiologically impossible for many women. I have seen women suffering both Type A and Type D symptoms in the same cycle, for example, so it is hard to see logically how the hormone imbalances can fit that picture: women can't have progesterone levels that are simultaneously too high and too low. In fact, many women have symptoms from each of Abraham's four groups during any one cycle. And for some women these can occur some months but not others. Some symptoms can also be more severe during some cycles.

Symptoms can also vary in how soon they hit each month. One woman might find that her mood swings escalate gradually, so that she feels more and more irritable up to the point when her period begins. Another can wake up one morning in mid-cycle and know instantly that she feels different – she'll be feeling tense or sad before she's even started the day. Partners of women with PMS have often remarked that they can see the difference first thing in the morning, because they see an altered person when they look into their eyes.

The bottom line is that many women suffer their own individual and unique group of symptoms from each of the four groups, at varying degrees and with varying regularity. All this makes Abraham's system of limited use. But this variability of symptoms does make one thing clear. Each sufferer from PMS has her own unique combination of symptoms, and this means any treatment will have to be tailor-made for her. Scientists simply aren't going to find one hormone treatment that will work for every woman, nor a single nutrient, such as magnesium, that will eliminate the problem.

Simply put, PMS symptoms are caused by a woman's negative response to changes in her hormonal cycle. One study found that using drugs to 'shut down' the monthly cycle eliminated all symptoms. When hormones – either oestrogen or progesterone – were added back, the symptoms returned immediately.[8] The only way to eliminate PMS permanently is to change our bodies at a fundamental level, so that when we go through the monthly cycle, our hormones work exactly as nature intended, and their natural shifts do not disrupt how we think or feel.

Risk factors

Who gets PMS? You are more likely to suffer from it if:

- You are in your thirties or forties
- You have two or more children
- Your mother suffered from it
- You have recently experienced a hormonal upheaval – for example, had a baby, a termination, miscarriage or sterilisation, or have stopped taking the Pill
- You have experienced several pregnancies in quick succession.

Remember that these are only risk factors. They are not set in stone. Research indicates that women who fall into these categories *could* be more likely to develop premenstrual symptoms. Unfortunately, the risk does appear to increase if you slot into more than one category. But knowing these risk factors can be helpful. If you know that you are at more risk than other women, it may spur you on to do something about it before your symptoms become worse.

It has been found that PMS can become increasingly worse as we age, and, as we saw above, that women in their thirties and forties can experience the most severe symptoms. My opinion is that as we get older our bodies have to work harder to deal with hormonal changes that occur naturally during the cycle, and that we also become more sensitive to these fluctuations. We also tend to have more responsibilities when we're older, leading to more stress. And if we're busier we may eat on the run, or erratically, skipping meals here and there. Thus our hormones can become unbalanced, giving rising to PMS.

Although it has been found that PMS has an inherited link, it's important to remember that this isn't a curse. Every woman is different, and how you look after yourself, how well you eat, how much and well you sleep, exercise and cope with stress, for example, will make a big difference not only to your overall health, but to how much you suffer from PMS.

The other risk factors are all linked to hormonal changes, such as having a baby. The recommendations in this book are designed to help your body deal with any hormonal fluctuations you have experienced in order to reduce premenstrual symptoms. While periods of change can be a major risk factor, it's something that you can control. In Chapter 6, you'll find out how.

Links with postnatal depression

You may ask what postnatal depression (PND) is doing in a book on PMS. As odd as it may sound, there is a connection. Dr Katharina Dalton has found that PMS sufferers – who normally feel exceptionally well during pregnancy, because they are not experiencing a cycle – have a higher risk of developing PND after the birth. In a nutshell, this means that if you are planning a pregnancy or suffered from PND following a previous pregnancy, you should take steps now to eliminate PMS, which will help to prevent a recurrence of PND.

PND is also known as the 'baby blues', and as postnatal illness or PNI, as depression is only one of the symptoms. It's very common and may occur on the day of the birth, the day after or even days later. Most women who suffer from it feel tearful and confused, symptoms partly caused by hormone changes during labour. The symptoms of PND can also be connected to hormonal disruptions that happen when the milk comes through. But for some 15 per cent of women, the despair and weeping persist, and develop into postnatal depression.

The symptoms of PND can include:

• Mood swings
• Comfort eating
• Crying
• Feelings of despair
• Exhaustion
• Feelings of inability to cope with the baby.

As you can see, these are very similar to some PMS symptoms.

If you had PND after an earlier pregnancy, chances are you could have it again – it happens in 68 per cent of cases. The hormonal changes you go through just after childbirth are a fairly major shock to the system, and your body needs to be balanced enough to cope with them to prevent any severe mental and physical symptoms.

There is also a very extreme form of PND called puerperal psychosis. This severe mental disorder is thankfully very rare. Women suffering from puerperal psychosis generally have to be hospitalised to prevent self-harm or harm to the baby. Depression is not the only symptom; irritability, hallucinations, confusion and anxiety may also set in after the birth.

Just as with PMS, the key to preventing PND is to work towards achieving optimum health, a big part of which is eating well. With PMS this allows your hormones to work correctly and your body to cope with their natural fluctuations month by month. With PND, it means your body will be able to weather the tremendous changes that happen during pregnancy and birth.

The severest symptoms

In 30 to 40 per cent of the women who suffer from PMS, symptoms can be serious enough to disrupt day-to-day life. The negative effects on family life, partners and children can be so powerful that these women describe a 'Jekyll and Hyde' change of which they are conscious but which they are unable to control. Some women with very severe PMS have experienced personality changes so extreme that they have committed murder or suicide in the weeks leading up to a period. Others have a specialised form of PMS that resembles severe depression (see page 15).

In 1981, one woman used the diagnosis of severe PMS as defence in a criminal case. After an argument with her boyfriend, this woman killed him by running him down with her car. The diagnosis of PMS was accepted on the grounds of diminished responsibility, and she claimed that she had 'just snapped'. She was given a conditional discharge for twelve months and banned from driving for twelve months.

Dr Katharina Dalton has often been an expert witness in legal cases involving PMS, and she cites a number of characteristics of PMS-related offences. They tend to be:

- recurrent offences
- without an accomplice
- not premeditated
- motiveless
- with no attempt to escape detection
- possibly a *cri de cœur* – a passionate appeal.

Dr Dalton explains that PMS cannot be used as a defence, but as a mitigating factor. This means that the woman must plead guilty but that PMS used in mitigation may change the sentencing.[9]

PMS has now been cited as a factor causing diminished responsibility in three murder trials, and has also been used as mitigation in cases of infanticide, baby-battering, arson, assault, damage to property, shoplifting, dangerous driving, hoax telephone calls and theft. What is important here is that although PMS must be recognised as an illness and women suffering from it do require treatment, it should not be used as a excuse for 'getting away with murder'. Dr Dalton says that the majority of women who break the law, claiming to have PMS, are found not to have the condition.

Although we tend to think of domestic violence as wife-battering, there are many men who are at the receiving end of both physical and verbal abuse from their partners. These men have described the violence as being entirely unpremeditated and unprovoked. Many men have described a scenario – often just a trivial argument or disagreement on a small point – in which only the slightest thing will set off a chain of fury and abuse, including kicking, punching, verbal insults and unbelievable violence. The most telling admission is that during pregnancy, all the violence and shouting stopped. PMS was undoubtedly implicated here.

Tragically, suicide is equally common in women with very severe PMS. Dr Dalton looked at the number of acute psychiatric hospital admissions and found that 53 per cent of the attempted suicides were admitted between the twenty-fifth day of their cycle and the fourth day of their next cycle. What's more, 47 per cent of admissions for depression occurred over those same days.[10]

Dr Dalton has also correlated the effect of PMS on accident rates,[11] as well as the effects of the menstrual cycle on a woman's family, by examining the number of hospital admissions for her children.[12] She found that women are more accident-prone during the days leading up to their periods, and that a normally vigilant and alert mother, who could anticipate and prevent a child's accident, can be more tired during the premenstrual days –

which increases the number of times her children must be admitted to hospital after accidents.

Premenstrual dysphoric disorder

In a small proportion of women – between 2 and 9 per cent – symptoms are very extreme, and destructive. This most severe form of premenstrual symptoms has its own name: premenstrual dysphoric disorder, or PMDD. The American Psychiatric Association Task Force has classed PMDD as a 'depressive disorder not otherwise specified' in *The Diagnostic and Statistical Manual of Mental Disorders* (4th edition).

The symptoms of PMDD strongly resemble deep depression. The main difference is that they occur only in the days leading up to the period. To be classed as suffering from PMDD, a woman must experience at least five of eleven specific symptoms, which include depressed mood, anxiety or tension, mood swings, irritability, lack of energy, change in appetite, sleep difficulties, feeling overwhelmed or out of control, and physical symptoms such as breast tenderness. Although PMDD covers literally dozens of physical symptoms, these are, for the purposes of diagnosis, considered a single symptom. The symptoms must be confirmed over two consecutive menstrual cycles. Quality of life is seriously affected in the second half of the cycle.

It has been suggested that PMDD is very different from other mood disorders, such as depression, for a number of reasons:

- The symptoms are cyclical – that is, they occur in an on-off pattern. 'Normal' depression is usually long-term (it lasts for weeks, months or even years), while the depression associated with PMDD lasts for about fourteen days at the most per month.
- The physical symptoms that accompany the mood changes are unique, and not characteristic of any other type of depression. The most common of these are breast tenderness and bloating.
- Appetite increases, and may include cravings for sweets. In most other kinds of depression there is a loss of appetite. Sex drive may increase – in rare cases, to the point of being classed as premenstrual nymphomania. In most cases of depression, there is little or no desire for sex.
- Weight increases. Most sufferers from depression lose weight.

So this is what we know about PMS. It hits in the days leading up to menstruation, and can vary in length from woman to woman. The severity of symptoms varies enormously, from mild to suicidal or violent. But after nearly seventy years of research, we're not much closer to pinpointing the cause of PMS. In the next section we look at the different theories and the mystery surrounding this condition.

CHAPTER 2

The Cause of PMS

The search for the root cause of PMS may not have got there yet – but it has inspired a number of theories. According to which study you read, the cause can include:

- Too much oestrogen in relation to progesterone
- Too much progesterone in relation to oestrogen
- Problems with glucose tolerance
- Too little serotonin
- Too much serotonin
- Too much adrenaline
- Low thyroid function
- An excess of androgens
- Not enough essential fatty acids
- An inherited problem
- Excess prolactin levels
- A vitamin B6 deficiency
- A magnesium deficiency
- Stress.

The difficulty in homing in on that one elusive cause stems from the fact that there is no laboratory test that can diagnose PMS, largely because the symptoms and potential causes vary so much between women. In some studies on women with PMS, researchers have found a deficiency or an excess of a particular hormone. In other studies, those deficiencies or excesses are not seen. Obviously, if a particular hormone was involved in PMS, we would expect to see it in every case of PMS. But we don't. What's more, although a number of hormones have been seen as a possible culprit – including oestrogen, androgens, progesterone and even adrenaline – some women do not have too much or too little of these hormones or, indeed, any notable hormone imbalances whatsoever.

PMS is, however, definitely linked to the menstrual cycle. Symptoms disappear if a woman is not ovulating (although she may still be having periods; see page 26), is pregnant or has had a hysterectomy with removal of the ovaries.[1]

Let's take a look at the different theories.

Too much oestrogen in relation to progesterone

In some of the studies it has been found that women with PMS have a mild progesterone deficiency and a mild excess of oestrogen.[2] This hormonal imbalance is thought to trigger PMS symptoms.

Too much progesterone in relation to oestrogen

It is now being suggested that having too much progesterone in relation to oestrogen could also cause PMS.[3] Studies have shown that using oestrogen to correct this imbalance has been effective.[4]

Problems with glucose tolerance

This theory has been suggested because of symptoms such as increased appetite and cravings for sweets and chocolate. Women with PMS have been found to have high abnormal glucose tolerance curves (or blood sugar imbalances), which could cause the shifts in appetite.[5]

Too little serotonin

Research has shown that blood levels of serotonin (the 'feelgood' brain chemical) are lower in some women with PMS.[6] When these women are given the SSRI family of antidepressants – selective serotonin re-uptake inhibitors, which include Prozac – the symptoms improve.

Too much serotonin

Other theories claim that too much serotonin can also be the cause of PMS, because if serotonin is too high it can give rise to nervousness, water retention, drowsiness and lack of concentration.[7]

Too much adrenaline

In response to stress, the adrenal glands produce higher levels of adrenaline. These glands use progesterone as the 'raw material' for producing adrenal hormones. If more adrenaline is produced, more progesterone is needed. So excessive adrenaline production can create a hormone imbalance where oestrogen is dominant.

Low thyroid function

Some studies have shown that a large proportion of women with PMS have low thyroid function (hypothyroidism).[8] Other research has shown hypothyroidism to be only slightly more common in these women.[9]

Symptoms of low thyroid function can include depression and fatigue, which can obviously be confused with PMS symptoms. Thyroid function is discussed in detail on pages 159–62. It's worth having your thyroid checked if you are experiencing what you think are PMS symptoms.

An excess of androgens

Some research has shown that women with premenstrual irritability and mood swings have higher levels of androgens (male hormones) than women without PMS, which could explain the symptoms.[10]

Not enough essential fatty acids

A lack of essential fatty acids (EFAs), present in oily fish and some nuts and seeds, has been suggested as the cause of PMS. The reason for this is that such a deficiency can cause problems with prostaglandins (see pages 60–1), hormone-like substances made from essential fatty acids. One important prostaglandin, PGE1, has a balancing effect on blood sugar and helps with water retention.

An inherited problem

This theory suggests that a woman has a genetic disposition towards having PMS because it 'runs in the family'.[11] It seems that you have a greater risk of having PMS if your mother also had it.

Excess prolactin levels

Prolactin is a hormone produced by the pituitary gland and released in high quantities when women are breastfeeding. The theory goes that if breast tenderness is one of a woman's PMS symptoms, she might have high levels of prolactin, although treatment with a drug that reduces prolactin levels has not been effective in the general treatment of PMS.

A vitamin B6 deficiency

Many studies have shown that PMS can be treated successfully with vitamin B6. So it would seem to follow that a deficiency of vitamin B6 can cause PMS. But, unfortunately, as in the majority of PMS studies, there is no definite proof. Some studies have shown that women with PMS are deficient in B6.[12] Others show no such deficiency.[13]

A magnesium deficiency

A number of studies have shown that magnesium supplements help with premenstrual symptoms, especially anxiety, tension and headaches.

Magnesium can be a bit tricky to test for. When testing for a deficiency, it is more accurate to look at magnesium levels in the red blood cells, rather than the serum (the liquid left after whole blood has been separated into its solid and liquid parts). Yet the normal procedure is to test the serum. So, part of the time, the accuracy of the testing could be suspect. Indeed, it's hard to know whether a deficiency of a particular nutrient or hormone would actually show up if the wrong part of the blood is analysed.

Keeping this in mind, the relevant research has been variable. Some shows that women with PMS have lower levels of red blood cell magnesium than women who don't suffer symptoms.[14] However, when serum levels of magnesium of women with PMS were examined, no deficiency of magnesium was found.[15]

Stress

Stress has been cited as a cause of PMS because it affects the functioning of the adrenal glands, which produce a number of hormones. One of these hormones, aldosterone, acts on the kidneys to regulate water balance. Another group of hormones produced by the adrenal glands, the glucocorticoids, help to regulate glucose metabolism. If this becomes unbalanced, changes in appetite and cravings for sweet foods can result.

Levels of one of the glucocorticoids, cortisol, can rise too high in very stressful situations, or when we do not cope well with stress. High levels of cortisol can trigger a number of symptoms, including depression, nervousness and insomnia, all similar to premenstrual symptoms. High levels of this hormone can also reduce the level of serotonin (see page 18), a condition that has also been suggested as a cause of PMS.

The real cause

As you'll have seen from the above, rooting out the cause of PMS has unearthed a mass of very different, and often conflicting, theories. We have a situation where one theory claims that PMS is caused by a deficiency of a particular hormone, while another says that an excess of that same hormone is actually the problem.

To add to the mystery, a very interesting experiment was published in the *New England Journal of Medicine* in 1998. The drug leuprolide, which switches off the sex hormones, was given to two groups of women. One group of women suffered regularly from PMS, and researchers found that their symptoms disappeared while taking the drug. The other group of women did not suffer from PMS. Both groups of women were given either oestrogen, progesterone or a placebo, and then asked to rate their symptoms. It was found that it didn't matter which hormone was given to the women with PMS – their symptoms returned within two weeks of taking the hormone. The non-PMS group reported no change. Even more confusingly, researchers found absolutely no difference between the hormone levels of either group. The conclusion was that although the female sex hormones need to be present to trigger PMS symptoms, they are not the cause of the problem.[16] It seems that it is a woman's individual response to the hormones that causes her to suffer the symptoms of PMS, not the hormones themselves.

This theory is also confirmed by looking at women from the Far East. Although they have the same circulating female hormones that we do, they do not suffer the same degree of premenstrual symptoms. It's obviously not the hormones that are at the root of the problem, but the way our bodies respond to them. That's why looking for a specific hormonal problem, or manipulating the cycle, is never going to be the long-term answer to PMS. The solution must be to address what the body is doing to cause these symptoms to emerge.

CHAPTER 3

Diagnosing PMS

We've seen how PMS defies testing by normal medical means. This is one of the toughest problems in dealing with the condition, and is one reason why experts across the years have insisted that it has no physical foundation, and is 'all in the mind'. Many women with suspected PMS are shunted from one specialist to another. Their blood tests look normal, but there is no question that they feel unwell – often desperately so – for weeks of every month.

A survey published in 1998 showed in the majority of cases, women have had to seek help from at least three different doctors for over five years before a diagnosis of PMS is made. And when the women studied did finally receive treatment, only 26 per cent of them were given a treatment that actually alleviated their symptoms. These women reported that 71 per cent of the doctors they visited were not adequately informed to diagnose and treat them, and only 23 per cent of them used a menstrual chart, which is currently the only way to confirm a PMS diagnosis. What's more, 76 per cent of the women in this survey said that they were not initially diagnosed by a doctor, but after they themselves suggested that they had PMS, the doctor agreed.[1]

Doctors are taught at medical school to diagnose by symptoms. PMS is being misdiagnosed – and persistently so – because doctors are looking at the *nature* of the symptoms, rather than the *timing* of those symptoms which is, of course, the key to PMS.

Of course, it is important to eliminate every other possible cause of symptoms before labelling anyone with PMS. In a way, this method is a sort of diagnosis by exclusion – once everything else can be ruled out, you are left with a diagnosis that can cover all sorts of female, cycle-related symptoms. Certainly problems such as anaemia, diabetes, thyroid conditions, endometriosis, depression and anxiety disorders share many symptoms with PMS, and must be ruled out and/or treated before PMS can be diagnosed. However, a simple menstrual chart (see opposite) will undoubtedly offer a clear picture of what's going on. That's where doctors are failing to address the obvious, by choosing to diagnose in a roundabout and often invasive fashion.

The *only* way to diagnose PMS with any accuracy is to write a menstrual diary. That means noting your symptoms on a daily basis, which will allow you to look for a pattern. The important factor is not what symptoms you have, but when they are occurring in the month. Later in this chapter I will explain an easy way to do this. But first let's look at what could be happening in your cycle, as this will help you understand the importance of timing in PMS.

A normal female hormone cycle

The first day of your period is also the first day of your next menstrual cycle. On this day, follicle-stimulating hormone (FSH) is released from your pituitary gland.

FSH triggers the growth of a group of follicles, or sacs, on the surface of the ovary. These follicles will eventually produce eggs.

Over the next two weeks (known as the 'follicular phase' of the menstrual cycle), the eggs grow and mature. At the same time, oestrogen levels, which are governed by the ovaries, begin to rise.

The pituitary gland then begins producing less FSH. Another hormone, luteinising hormone or LH, is galvanised into action. LH is also produced by the pituitary gland. Fertile alkaline mucus is produced in the cervix; this provides the right conditions to keep sperm alive, and to encourage their movement through the cervix and up towards the fallopian tubes, where fertilisation – if any – takes place.

The surge in LH causes ovulation: a mature egg (normally only one, but sometimes more) is released from a follicle and enters the fallopian tube.

The empty follicle becomes known as the corpus luteum, and it begins to produce a hormone known as progesterone. The second half of the cycle (called the luteal phase) has begun.

If fertilisation occurs, the fertilised egg will travel down the fallopian tube and implant in the lining of the womb (known as the endometrium).

If fertilisation does not occur, the lining of the womb breaks down and is

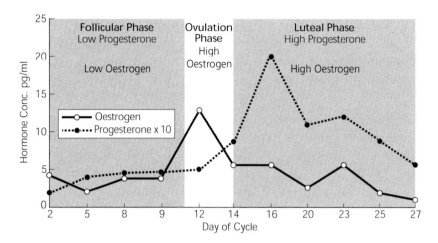

A normal female hormonal cycle

expelled in your normal monthly period. At the same time, there is a rapid and dramatic fall in the levels of oestrogen and progesterone. This drop in hormone levels signals the start of the next cycle.

To give you a clear idea of how hormone levels rise and fall over a monthly cycle, I have also written them down in 'days', so that you can match them up with the diagram. Remember that we are all unique, so these days are only rough guides to what will actually take place. Some women will have short cycles, some long cycles, and some will have cycles that vary from month to month.

Days 1–4   Period starts. Low oestrogen with rising levels of FSH
Days 5–8   Rising oestrogen levels
Days 9–12   Peak oestrogen levels
Days 13–16 Ovulation, peak levels of LH and FSH, and fairly high oestrogen, but below peak level
Days 17–20 Post-ovulation, with lower oestrogen and rising progesterone
Days 21–24 High progesterone and high oestrogen
Days 25–28 Falling progesterone, if there is no pregnancy, and falling oestrogen

> **CAN YOU HAVE A PERIOD AND NOT OVULATE?**
> Many women will not ovulate during a cycle, and may be unaware of this fact, unless they are normally aware of ovulation taking place. Some women, for example, will experience a sharp pain in the region of the ovaries (just above the pubic bone), along with a change in cervical mucus, during ovulation.
>
> Ovulation without periods becomes more common as a woman approaches the menopause, or where there is a hormone imbalance and the egg is not being released. When ovulation does not take place, the hormone progesterone is not produced in that cycle. So just because you are having periods does not automatically mean that you are ovulating.

Second half of the cycle (luteal phase)

PMS occurs in the second half of your cycle – the so-called luteal phase – and at one time, the extreme symptoms of PMS were called 'late luteal phase dysphoric disorder'. Quite a mouthful!

Because the symptoms take place in the second half of the cycle, one of the main focuses has been on progesterone, because it is only released during this phase. The general consensus (although the PMS specialist Dr Katharina Dalton would disagree) is that if women are not ovulating – and that includes those women who are still having periods without ovulation – they do not suffer the symptoms of PMS. In those cycles, oestrogen will be produced without progesterone. But hormone profiles of women with PMS have not shown conclusive results. Neither the oestrogen nor the progesterone levels of women with PMS differ from those of women without PMS.[2] What's more, neither the timing nor the severity of the symptoms correlates with fluctuations in hormone levels in individual women.[3]

Hormones: the inside story

We've seen how intimately involved in PMS hormones are. Now it's time to take a closer look at these important actors in the drama.

The word 'hormone' comes from the Greek for 'urge on'. And that's precisely what they do. These chemical messengers, which are carried in the blood, trigger activity in different organs and parts of the body.

The reproductive hormones control your monthly cycle, and help to maintain pregnancy. The hypothalamus in the brain releases a hormone called gonadotrophin-releasing hormone (GnRH) in small amounts every 90 minutes. This pulsing effect releases both FSH and LH from the pituitary gland. The pituitary gland controls the release of both FSH and LH, which then triggers the production of hormones by the ovaries. The pituitary gland also releases TSH (thyroid-stimulating hormone), which in turn helps to control the normal functioning of the thyroid gland. The thyroid hormones control your metabolism and your body temperature. The adrenal glands produce hormones that help you to cope with stress, and others that regulate fat, protein and carbohydrate metabolism. Your adrenals also produce a hormone called aldosterone, which acts on the kidneys to regulate water balance. And your pancreas secretes the hormone insulin, which regulates the amount of sugar (glucose) in your blood.

The 'conductor'

It has been suggested that the 'conductor' or regulator of this intricate system is the hypothalamus, which is found in the brain. This gland contains several centres that control body temperature, thirst, hunger and eating, water balance and sexual function. It is also closely connected with sleeping and waking (like an internal body clock), and has a direct or indirect effect on the ovaries, adrenal glands, thyroid, breasts and kidneys.

The hypothalamus may control all the different parts of the body, but it operates by feedback. The mechanism is similar to the thermostat on a central heating system. In this case the thermostat (the hypothalamus) will switch on the heating system (all the endocrine glands) when the temperature in the house (the body) drops too low, and then when it registers that the temperature is at a good level, it switches it off again. Unfortunately, the situation can arise where there is nothing wrong with the central heating system, but the thermostat is malfunctioning, so it can seem like the heating is not working properly. For example, if the hypothalamus, whch helps to control appetite, is malfunctioning, it takes longer than usual for you to get the message that you have eaten enough. During that delay, you were not feeling 'full' or 'satisfied' and carried on eating more than was appropriate. Over time, this would then effect your weight.

Or, taking it further, you could have a situation where somebody turns on an electric heater while the central heating is on. Because extra heat is being supplied from outside the central heating system, the thermostat registers the temperature increases and switches itself off. This is similar to taking hormones in the form of the contraceptive Pill which mimics the hormonal state of pregnancy. The hypothalamus is functioning normally, but it registers that you are 'pregnant' and so it doesn't send the message down to the ovaries that it's time to ovulate. You can't get pregnant because your body thinks you already are.

The perfect balance

It's fairly clear that every system in your body is dependent on every other system. Nothing works or operates in isolation. Therefore, an imbalance of any sort – hormonal, nutritional, or even stress- or sleep-related – could have a profound effect. And that's just one of the reasons why it is so important to be treated holistically – as a 'whole' person, rather than a collection of separate systems and symptoms. This interrelation of systems is clearly seen in PMS. I suggest that's why the conventional search for one cause and one treatment for PMS has been so unsuccessful: each woman is unique, with a unique balance of physical systems.

It is possible to treat PMS and to eliminate it completely. However, in order for this to happen, past methods of looking at and dealing with PMS have to be turned on their heads. So far, most researchers have looked at this condition from the wrong direction.

> **OESTROGEN**
> Oestrogen is not one hormone, but several hormones grouped together under the one name. They include oestradiol, oestriol and oestrone. For the sake of clarity, I will use the term oestrogen to mean all of them collectively.
>
> Oestrogen is the key hormone responsible for ensuring that a woman matures from childhood through to adulthood. It causes the breasts to develop and helps produce the characteristic feminine shape.

The menstrual diary

There are many different charts that have been used to monitor PMS symptoms. Some are very time-consuming to fill out, demanding that you work your way through up to forty different symptoms per day, rating each symptom according to its severity on a scale from 1 to 3. This kind of chart also makes it complicated to look for a pattern of symptoms through the month.

One of the best methods for charting symptoms was devised by Dr Katharina Dalton, who has tried to make the whole process easy to complete and easy to read afterwards.

Here's how it works. First, consider the three symptoms that affect you the most, or cause the most discomfort or inconvenience. Say, for example, you choose headaches, irritability and breast tenderness. Give each of them a letter, such as, H = headaches, I = irritability and B = breast tenderness. You use capital letters (H, I, B) when the symptoms are severe, and lower-case letters (h, i, b) when the symptoms are mild.

Then choose a symbol or letter to represent your periods (such as P, M or even X). At the end of each day, fill in the chart and list what symptoms, if any, you have experienced that day. So, on one day, for example, you may put an 'h' if you had a mild headache, 'B' if your breasts felt very uncomfortable, but no 'I' because you didn't feel irritable. Some women like to put a small dot in the box at the end of a day with no symptoms at all, so that they know that they did remember to complete the chart.

You need to complete the chart for at least two consecutive menstrual cycles to get a clear picture of what is happening.

This method of charting makes it easy to see the pattern of symptoms through the month. It is also excellent when you start to make some of the changes recommended in this book. If you carry on completing the charts, you will be able to make an accurate comparison of a 'before' and an 'after' picture of your symptoms.

It is no good trying to sort out your premenstrual symptoms retrospectively – in other words, it won't help to work out at the end of the month how you felt and what symptoms you experienced. Menstrual charting for the diagnosis of PMS must be done on a daily basis. Our memories are very selective; some women can 'forget' symptoms, whereas others exaggerate them. Some women have come to see me about headaches along with other health problems. At a follow-up consultation I have asked them how they are progressing and they relay what symptoms have improved. When I ask about the headaches, they often pause before realising that they have disappeared completely. Without the pain present, they've forgotten. It's easy to forget symptoms that come and go on a daily, weekly or even monthly basis, which is why it is so important to fill in the chart every day, whether a symptom is there or not.

When you start looking for a pattern, you'll need to analyse the chart. Do your symptoms start in the week or so leading up to your period and then stop almost immediately when you bleed? If so, you have PMS. You should have almost a week free of symptoms before they start again.

You may be surprised to see, as you watch your charts develop over a two-month period or longer, that there are, literally, great chunks of your life where you are not feeling entirely well. You could be having two weeks of premenstrual symptoms, one week of bleeding with your period, and only seven days of feeling 'normal'. In real terms, this means that you are feeling well for only a quarter of the month, which is really only a quarter of your life. The other three-quarters is governed by your cycle. Luckily, that's something that can be changed.

CHAPTER 4

The Conventional Approach to PMS

In this chapter we'll be looking at the conventional approach to PMS. How does this variable and elusive condition fare in the medical context?

As we've seen, the problem with the medical approach to PMS is twofold. First, for treatment to be offered, a diagnosis must be made. We discussed the drawbacks of the conventional system of diagnosing this condition in Chapter 3, and also pointed out that this process can take as long as five years. What's more, if the doctor has failed to pinpoint what's causing a woman's PMS, any treatment they offer is unlikely to be successful in the long term. Many women will have to contend with a hit-and-miss round of differing treatments offered over a long period of time.

In their search for causes, some doctors have homed in on the fact that when women do not have female sex hormones circulating around their bodies, they do not suffer the symptoms of PMS. Thus the most popular treatment to date has aimed to shut off the female hormones, in order to prevent the symptoms from occurring.

Other treatments have tried to treat individual symptoms. One medical paper suggested diuretics for water retention, bromocriptine, danazol or tamoxifen (see below) for breast tenderness, and diphenhydramine for sleep disturbances. This is a potentially powerful cocktail of drugs, and could cause side-effects as debilitating as the symptoms of PMS themselves.

On the other hand, because some symptoms of PMS can be predominately psychological, including depression, mood swings and irritability, tranquillisers or antidepressants can be prescribed. In fact, the latest research seems to indicate antidepressants as the primary treatment for PMS (see pages 41–2). This approach undoubtedly relieves some women's psychological symptoms. But remember that PMS affects you for only part of the month – so you could be taking strong drugs the whole month for a problem that is there for only a few days.

The most important drawback to all this, however, is that conventional medication focuses on relieving symptoms. It does not ultimately address or change the underlying cause of PMS, and it only works while you are taking the medication. The moment you stop, the symptoms return.

Finally, there are still many doctors who do not view PMS as a health problem, and some women have been told to 'grin and bear it' as part and parcel of being a woman.[1] This a potentially dangerous attitude: women who are clearly in distress are being ignored. Not only that, but it can become a self-fulfilling prophecy – women suffering from PMS begin to believe that they are imagining it all, and that there is something psychologically wrong with them. Quite apart from that, because it can take many years before these women are given the treatment they need to alleviate the problem once and for all, they can end up having to cope with a very poor quality of life for a long time.

Drugs

Generally speaking, drugs are used in two ways: either to shut down female hormones, manipulating the different hormones during a cycle to see whether there is an improvement in the symptoms; or to treat specific symptoms, such as water retention, breast tenderness or depression.

The Pill

The Pill works as a contraceptive because it prevents ovulation, alters the lining of the womb, and makes the mucus in the cervix hostile to sperm, should ovulation occur. The hormones in it are a combination of synthetic oestrogen and progestogen. They are taken for three weeks and then stopped for a week. The bleeding that women on the Pill experience is not an actual period but simply a 'withdrawal bleed' that comes on when the synthetic hormones are stopped. There are a number of Pill formulations with differing hormone combinations and strengths.

When the Pill has been used to treat PMS, results have been mixed. It seems to work for some women, but others find that it makes the problem worse. On balance, research shows that the Pill is not effective in treating

PMS.[2] In fact, some women who do not normally suffer from PMS will experience symptoms for the first time when they start taking the Pill – an obvious reason to stop taking it immediately.

It's the progestogen part of the Pill that often causes the most problems. Some recorded side-effects of the Pill are nausea, vomiting, headaches, thrombosis, changes in sex drive, depression and breast tenderness. Of course, many of these are also premenstrual symptoms, so for some women it exacerbates existing problems, and for others creates PMS-like symptoms where none existed previously. Some women are less susceptible to the side-effects of the Pill, so preventing ovulation can help their PMS symptoms.

Recently, in a report in the *Lancet*, it was suggested that if women are given the Pill continuously, without their week's respite every month, their hormone cycles can be controlled.[3] This could be a major change in lifestyle and possibly in health, as women today menstruate nearly three times as much as previous generations. As we saw earlier, this is because they now choose to have fewer children and do not breastfeed for as long, which increases the number of periods. This report in the *Lancet* suggested that women should have the right to choose whether or not to have periods! If you take the Pill continuously, you could end up eliminating your periods for ever. Nobody knows what the long-term effects of controlling the cycle like this would be.

GnRH (gonadotrophin-releasing hormone) analogues

GnRH is a type of medication that includes buserelin and goserelin, and stops the normal menstrual cycle by plunging you into a temporary menopause. It's made up of synthetic hormones – 'analogue', meaning 'similar', denotes the fact that they're synthetic – that can be given as an injection or a nasal spray.

In a normal cycle, as we've seen, GnRH is released naturally from the hypothalamus in the brain in small amounts every ninety minutes. This pulsing effect in turn releases both FSH and LH from the pituitary gland. This synthetic treatment gives a constant dose to the hypothalamus, which stops the pituitary from releasing both FSH and LH. The production of hormones by the ovaries is then halted, thereby preventing ovulation. Unfortunately, the symptoms of the menopause, such as hot flushes and night sweats, can be as debilitating as PMS. There are also concerns about the long-term use (over six months) of these drugs, and they carry an increased risk of osteoporosis because they give you low levels of oestrogen.

Other side-effects of synthetic GnRH include breakthrough bleeding, headaches, nausea, mood changes such as depression, breast tenderness, abdominal pain, fatigue, weight changes, nervousness, dizziness, drowsiness, acne, dry skin, back pain, muscle pain, ovarian cysts, skin rashes, constipation, vomiting, sleep disorders, blurred vision and changes in body hair. Many of these side-effects could be worse than the symptoms of PMS.

And because of the menopausal symptoms associated with these drugs, the conventional response has been to use 'add-back' regimes − in other words, to introduce some combination of oestrogen and progestogen to create an artificial hormonal environment that will minimise the side-effects of the GnRH analogues. But although this may protect you from osteoporosis and reduce side-effects such as hot flushes, it may aggravate the very PMS symptoms that the GnRH analogues are being taken to treat. Even more worryingly, some studies have found no improvement compared with the placebo when using this regime.[4] In particular, this type of treatment does not seem to help women with severe mood swings − one of the most debilitating symptoms of PMS. One study has shown that this 'add-back' therapy can help to reduce the symptoms of PMS,[5] but, once again, treatment is only effective for as long as the medication is taken.

There are further issues here. Taking these analogues halts the production of female hormones, which are then added back to control the resulting side-effects. Not only is this a serious disruption of natural body function, but it involves heavy long-term drug use, which can never be acceptable − particularly in the light of the fact that it does nothing to address the cause of the condition in the first place.

Danazol

Danazol is a synthetic weak male hormone that prevents ovulation and turns off ovarian function, which in turn stops periods. In essence it works on the same principle as the Pill and the GnRH analogues: it is believed that controlling the output of hormones from the ovaries can in turn control PMS symptoms. It does have a number of side-effects, including severe mood swings, nausea, dizziness, rashes and headaches and, because it is a mild male hormone, the growth of facial hair, acne, an increased sex drive, weight gain and deepening of the voice.

Because danazol shuts off ovarian function, the ovaries stop producing oestrogen, and other side-effects can arise which are similar to those of the menopause, including hot flushes and vaginal dryness. Male hormones have some protective effects against osteoporosis, so the risk is not the same as for women taking GnRH analogues. But there is no question that the additional symptoms brought on by this drug are more distressing than PMS.

Danazol has, however, been particularly effective in treating premenstrual migraines[6] and, when given only in the second half of the cycle, it has helped alleviate breast tenderness, but it has failed to have much effect on any other symptoms.[7] But research into the efficacy of this drug has been limited: not surprisingly, many women who took part in a study looking at the effects of danazol on PMS withdrew because of the side-effects.[8]

Like the women who left that study, you'd have to weigh up which symptoms are worse – those caused by the drug or the PMS. There are also much more natural ways of dealing with menstrual migraines and breast tenderness, making it clear that the risks could certainly not outweigh the benefits.

Bromocriptine

This drug works by reducing high levels of prolactin, the hormone that is released in high quantities when women are breastfeeding. Because of this link with the breasts, bromocriptine has been prescribed for women whose main premenstrual symptom is breast pain. In some cases, it has been effective. But women with breast tenderness do not necessarily have high prolactin levels. Bromocriptine has no effect on other premenstrual symptoms. It's a powerful drug with side-effects that can include nausea, vomiting, headaches and dizziness. In my opinion, it is too strong a treatment for breast tenderness or pain when there are much more natural ways of dealing with the symptoms.

Mefenamic acid

Mefenamic acid is usually used in the treatment of painful periods and heavy menstrual flow because it inhibits certain prostaglandins – the hormone-like substances that can be either harmful or beneficial to health. One particular prostaglandin (PGE2) is highly inflammatory, causing swelling and pain and, at high levels, also thickening the blood.

One theory suggests that PMS is caused by an excess of prostaglandins, and a number of studies have shown that if mefenamic is taken during the second half of the cycle, the results are better than the placebo.[9] But across the various studies, the drug alleviated a number of different symptoms. Mefenamic acid seems to help headaches, mood swings and breast pain, but it has had mixed results with symptoms such as irritability, tension and depression, some of the most common and serious problems women with PMS experience. The side-effects centre in the digestive tract and include indigestion, diarrhoea, nausea, abdominal cramps, constipation, bloating and flatulence. Therefore, at the moment, given the inconsistent results of the studies, it would not be a drug of choice for PMS.

Diuretics

Diuretics were one of the first treatments offered for PMS, and are still often used to help with water retention and weight gain before a period. They work by interfering with the normal action of the kidneys and so promoting the release of urine. Osmotic, loop and thiazide diuretics reduce the amount of sodium and water taken back into the blood, thus increasing the volume of urine. Other diuretics increase blood flow through the kidneys, and thus the amount of water they filter and expel in the urine.

Diuretics do increase the rate at which fluid is lost, but will also flush out important minerals. For example, more potassium can be excreted, which can be dangerous. One of the most important roles of potassium is to ensure that your heart functions correctly. In some cases, potassium salts are offered alongside diuretics, to avoid the loss of much of this key mineral.

One of the most effective diuretics used in the treatment of PMS is spironolactone. This works by blocking aldosterone – a hormone released by the adrenal glands – which acts on the kidneys to regulate water balance. Spironolactone is classed as a potassium-sparing diuretic, so it does not cause as much potassium loss as other diuretics.

Not all the research into the use of spironolactone for PMS is positive, but one trial showed that taking 100mg of the drug from day 14 until menstruation helped with water retention.[10] Although this was a double-blind placebo-controlled trial, because of the way a diuretic works, women involved in studies like this can tell whether they are taking the drug or the placebo. Obviously, they know when they are passing more urine! Someone passing more water will expect to feel less bloated, which would, of course, alter the result. For this reason, studies into the use of diuretics to treat premenstrual bloating are much more likely to be flawed, or at least not truly double-blind.

Diuretics will only help to ease water retention, not any of the other symptoms of PMS, and side-effects can include gastrointestinal disturbances, headaches, confusion, rashes and menstrual disturbances.

There are natural diuretics (see pages 113–14), which allow fluid to be released without your losing vital nutrients. These treatments are also free of side-effects. Changing your diet (see page Chapter 5) is also important, for not only does this ease the symptoms of PMS, including water retention, but it addresses the cause, so that it is dealt with once and for all.

Oestrogen

Taking oestrogen is another way of controlling the cycle by suppressing ovulation. Oestrogen patches or implants have been used in studies on PMS.

One study used 100mg implants of oestrogen, and the women in question were also given 5mg of a progestogen (noresthisterone) for seven days each month (to protect the womb lining from becoming too thick). The control group in this study were given placebo implants and placebo tablets. Those taking the placebo showed a 94 per cent improvement over the first two months of treatment.[11] Not surprisingly, this waned over time.

The oestrogen doses used in the study are extremely high for young women and no one knows the long-term effect of such a treatment. Doses of this level have in the past been given to menopausal women who have low oestrogen levels.

What is interesting about this study is that none of the women taking progestogen reported side-effects, while in the same year, a study by the same researchers, using the same progestogen with oestrogen implants for postmenopausal women, showed significant negative side-effects.[12]

One report commented on this discrepancy, suggesting that 'perhaps there were more disadvantages from the progestogens than were admitted in this report'[13] especially when these same researchers have shown that the side-effects caused by using progestogen alongside oestrogen implants have resulted in a high rate of hysterectomies.[14]

The hysterectomies were given for different reasons, for example prolapse and prolonged bleeding, even when adequate progestogens were given. In all cases of hysterectomy caused by this treatment, the women involved were found to have enlarged wombs.

Oestrogen patches (at 100mcg) have been shown to be effective in the treatment of PMS symptoms.[15] This type of treatment is the equivalent of using hormone replacement therapy (HRT) to treat premenstrual symptoms, and there are risks attached to taking HRT, such as breast cancer.

In the early part of 2000, two separate studies showed an increased risk of breast cancer in women taking HRT. One, from the *Journal of the American Medical Association*, studied over 46,000 women and found a 40 per cent increase in breast cancer risk in women taking HRT.[16] Other side-effects of HRT can include breast tenderness, bloating, depression, skin rashes, hair loss, thrush, womb cancer and weight changes. In my opinion, where there are natural ways of eliminating PMS, the risks of taking oestrogen don't outweigh the benefits.

Progesterone

This is the 'hot potato' of the PMS world. The use of progesterone for PMS has been very controversial, with arguments raging for and against this treatment. Progesterone is the hormone that is released after ovulation and because PMS obviously occurs in the second half of the cycle, it makes sense that progesterone might be at the root.

Dr Katharina Dalton pioneered the treatment of PMS with progesterone. It is normally given in the form of vaginal pessaries because when progesterone is given by mouth, it is rapidly broken down by the liver.

The arguments have centred around the fact that if extra progesterone needs to be given to eliminate PMS, then women with PMS must be deficient in it. But that is not the case. There are many studies that do not show reduced levels of progesterone in women with PMS.[17]

It has also been suggested that PMS may be caused not by an outright progesterone deficiency, but by an imbalance between oestrogen and progesterone – in other words, too much oestrogen in relation to progesterone. However, this theory has not been successfully proved either.[18]

Some of the confusion lies in the fact that the research on progesterone and progestogens (see page 40) has been 'lumped together'. These two substances are not the same, and should never be viewed as such. When used as a drug, progesterone is chemically similar to the hormone that is produced by the ovaries. Progestogens, however, are synthetic hormones. One type of progestogen, noresthisterone, is more similar to testosterone (the 'male' hormone) than it is to progesterone.

As with much of the other research on treatments for PMS, some studies show that progesterone works,[19] while others claim that it definitely doesn't. In some cases, the progesterone fared even worse than the placebo in clinical trials.[20]

Progesterone creams are also available for external use (on the skin), but doctors are not convinced that enough progesterone is absorbed this way. Progesterone in the form of pessaries and creams (for either the vagina or the skin) are classed as being 'natural' to distinguish it from the synthetic progestogens (see dydrogesterone below). But the word 'natural' used in front of progesterone is misleading. In this context, it simply means that the progesterone is chemically identical to that which you produce from your own ovaries. It is a hormone and it needs to be prescribed by a doctor.

Some progesterone creams are made from wild yam, which has intensi-fied the confusion surrounding the drug. Many women have been misled into believing that they are taking a herbal product in the form of an extract from the wild yam plant. They are not. Progesterone is synthesised from wild yam in a laboratory. Oestrogens can also be synthesised in a lab-oratory from wild yam or soya. Synthesising means making something that is chemically identical. It doesn't mean extracting a natural substance. Once again, you must remember that progesterone is a drug, not a herbal product.

Side-effects arising from progesterone, as listed in the *British National Formulary* – the reference book used by doctors to look up drugs – can include weight changes, acne, water retention, premenstrual symptoms, irregular menstrual cycles and breast discomfort. A number of women have reported to me that when they used the progesterone cream, their breasts actually seemed larger. Some studies have shown that progesterone may, in fact, be a risk factor for breast cancer.[21]

The pessary has been associated with further problems, including the possibility of a localised yeast infection (candidiasis), which can lead to itch-ing and irritation.

Progestogens

These are synthetic hormones that normally make up part of the combination contraceptive Pill. They work by making the mucus in the cervix hostile to sperm, and in some women they also inhibit ovulation.

There are two types of progestogens: the first group are analogues (meaning 'similar to') of progesterone (such as dydrogesterone and medroxyprogesterone), and the second are analogues of testosterone (such as norethisterone). Both types of progestogens are used in the Pill and, when stopped, cause a withdrawal bleed, or artificial period. They are also included in HRT medications in order to stop the womb lining from building up to excessive levels.

Dydrogesterone has been used in some studies on PMS. Once again, it has been shown to be effective in some studies and not others. The problem is that many women experience the symptoms of PMS when they begin taking these progestogens, for example as HRT.

The *British National Formulary* lists potential side-effects as: premenstrual symptoms, gastrointestinal disturbances, water retention, weight changes, breast discomfort, changes in libido, irregular menstrual cycles, depression and insomnia. Not a great trade-off, in my view.

What's more, recent research published in the *International Journal of Cancer*[22] has shown that one of the most potent angiogenesis factors now known in cancer research – VEGF, or vascular endothelial cell growth factor – is stimulated by progestogens. Angiogenesis is the process in which new blood vessels are formed. This process is essential for a tumour to develop, and we now know that it is promoted by VEGF. This may sound confusing, but it's really very simple. Progestogens are now known to increase the growth of new blood vessels that will allow a tumour to develop and grow. Dangerous business.

Tamoxifen

Women with breast cancer are treated with tamoxifen to prevent a recurrence of the disease. It works as an anti-oestrogen by blocking the oestrogen receptors in the breasts. Tamoxifen has been used to treat premenstrual breast problems. In the test it was taken from day 5 to day 24 of the cycle, and was reported to be effective.[23] One study claimed that 90 per cent of the women taking the drug reported that their symptoms had gone.

However, 86 per cent of the group taking the placebo in this study said they had also had a reduction in symptoms!

No one knows the long-term effects of taking a drug like tamoxifen. In the short term, it often causes uncomfortable side-effects that can resemble all the symptoms of the menopause, such as hot flushes and vaginal dryness. And many women who take tamoxifen find that their periods stop altogether. Young women taking this drug could be putting themselves at risk of osteoporosis, and there is also an increased risk of womb cancer. Although it blocks the oestrogen receptors in the breasts, tamoxifen can actually increase the risk of womb cancer. This can happen when it is picked up by receptors in the womb lining, as it can overstimulate them. Receptors are proteins that work like a lock; the hormones are the keys and fit into them. If the receptors are being overstimulated or bombarded, there is the potential for cancerous growth.

This is not a drug to use unless absolutely necessary – in the case of breast cancer, for example – and it's certainly not suitable for a premenstrual symptom such as breast pain, which can be treated effectively through natural means. Its benefits definitely do not outweigh the risks associated with it.

Antidepressants

Because one of the major symptoms of PMS is depression, it has been suggested that it be treated as a mental illness. As discussed in Chapter 1, some 5 per cent of all PMS sufferers have symptoms that are so severe during the second half of their cycle that their lives are completely disrupted. The condition is known as premenstrual dysphoric disorder or PMDD (see page 15). It has been suggested that antidepressants should be the first choice of treatment for sufferers of this serious condition.

However, a number of studies have looked at the effects of different antidepressants on PMS (not just PMDD), including tricyclic antidepressants such as amitriptyline, benzodiazepines and SSRIs (selective serotonin re-uptake inhibitors).

With the benzodiazepines, one in particular, alprazolam, has been shown to be effective in treating all the psychological symptoms of PMS.[24] Unfortunately, this drug is potentially addictive and there can be withdrawal symptoms when it is discontinued, including tremors, nausea, excess perspiration and muscle cramps – basically, it involves going 'cold turkey'.

Common side-effects are drowsiness and light-headedness, and it has not been demonstrated as being safe in pregnancy. Given that women experiencing PMS are still fertile, and have the potential to become pregnant, even by accident, it's worth noting the risks.

Because of these major drawbacks, other benzodiazepines have been substituted, but they do not give the same results in the treatment of PMS.

With the female hormone theory of PMS failing to gather adherents, the arguments have switched to looking at PMS as a problem with fluctuating levels of neurotransmitters, or brain chemicals. Serotonin, which acts as a neurotransmitter, is believed to have an important influence on mood, and levels have been shown to be different in women with PMS. In women without PMS, levels of serotonin rise in the second half, or luteal phase, of the cycle, and reach their peak just before the period. In women with PMS, the levels of serotonin appear to remain the same throughout the entire cycle.

SSRI antidepressants work by preventing the brain from absorbing serotonin, thereby maintaining adequate levels. Analytic research done in 2000, which looked at 101 previous studies, showed that SSRIs were effective in treating severe psychological symptoms of PMS even when taken only in the second half of the cycle.[25] Unfortunately, women taking the SSRIs were 2.5 times more likely to withdraw from the trials, and to stop taking medication, than those who were taking the placebo. The main reason was the side-effects, which include gastrointestinal disturbances, nausea, fatigue or lethargy, and insomnia.

The Psychopharmacologic Drugs Advisory Committee of the US Food and Drug Administration has voted to recommend that Prozac, or fluoxetine, which is an SSRI, be approved for the treatment of PMDD. If this goes ahead, Prozac will be first drug ever approved for PMDD. This is cause for some concern, as it could potentially be used in the general treatment of PMS. It is not yet known how effective SSRIs are for the physical symptoms of PMS because most of the trials with this type of antidepressant have involved women whose symptoms are mainly psychological. Furthermore, the wide-scale use of any drug for symptoms that are as varied as those associated with PMS is not advisable, particularly given the potential for dependency.

Surgery

Surgery is the most drastic treatment imaginable for PMS, but from a medical point of view, it is a viable option. A while back I was speaking at a conference on PMS, at the Medical Society, and one gynaecologist's talk involved 'treating' PMS with a total hysterectomy – that is, removing the ovaries as well as the womb. Not only is a total hysterectomy a shocking approach to a cyclical problem, but the womb would not even need to be removed to have an effect. It is really only the ovaries that are problematic in the case of PMS, because they produce the sex hormones. This is like taking drugs to shut down ovarian function – but never being able to stop. Don't even consider it. You would be plunged into a surgical menopause overnight and would effectively be replacing PMS with menopausal symptoms, as well as having the trauma of an operation to bear.

Conclusions on the conventional medical approach to PMS

The sheer number of different drugs on offer makes it fairly clear that there is a great deal of confusion about the medical approach to treating PMS. Some studies show that oestrogen works for PMS and others show that progesterone is the key. These are two completely different hormones that work in very different ways. It is virtually impossible that they could *both* work. Other studies state that neither oestrogen nor progesterone has any effect on PMS.

As I mentioned in the introduction to this section of the book, one of the most interesting aspects of PMS research is that there is an enormously high placebo effect. What this means is that people taking 'dummy' tablets, rather than a drug or anything else, often experience relief from symptoms. There are always some people in any study who will respond to the placebos, but in the case of PMS, it's 94 per cent of the participants![26]

Sometimes better results are obtained from the placebo than from the medication being tested. Because of this placebo effect, some say that PMS is all in the mind, and doesn't really exist as a physical condition. But other researchers have suggested that the placebo effect is important and should be studied in some detail to understand how and why it is occurring.

For instance, one way of looking at this phenomenon is that when women have been given an opportunity to talk and to have their symptoms taken seriously, these will improve whether they take drugs or a placebo. Too often symptoms are dismissed out of hand, and women may simply respond better to a different approach.

Remember, if you are going to take medication to treat PMS, such as

GnRH analogues or antidepressants, you will probably be taking that drug until you reach the menopause. Every time you stop the medication, your symptoms will return. These medications work by suppressing symptoms. No fundamental change in your body has occurred – but this is necessary if the problem is to be eliminated. When you reach the menopause, you will undoubtedly experience relief from PMS because your ovaries will eventually stop producing sex hormones. But if you begin taking HRT, not only might you experience side-effects, but the progestogens in that medication could reproduce the symptoms of PMS.

In the end, the real aim is to eliminate PMS by discovering why you have the symptoms in the first place. This is the only permanent solution. And in Part Two, we'll be exploring it in detail.

PART TWO

THE NATURAL APPROACH TO TREATING PMS

Introduction

When researchers compare the hormone levels of women with PMS and those without it, why can't they find a difference – particularly since PMS is so clearly linked to the menstrual cycle? It's actually quite simple. The *amount* (either excess or deficiency) of hormones is not the cause of PMS. The problem lies in the *way* your body responds to these hormones.

Consider this scenario: you are starving and are put into a room where there is plenty of food. But it's just out of arm's reach, and you are restrained in such a way that you cannot move to pick it up. The food is there, but you're barred from using it to nourish yourself. The same principle applies to your hormones. It doesn't matter how much you have of any particular hormones – if your body cannot utilise them, it's as bad as having none at all.

Now let's look at the symptoms. It is assumed that PMS affects a woman's general health by causing any combination of 150 different symptoms. But what if the situation is really the other way round? What, in other words, if your general health is what's causing PMS to manifest itself?

If you have not been eating well – perhaps failing to keep up your levels of certain vitamins and minerals – not exercising, suffering from stress and generally feeling run down, it is very possible that your body's ability to produce the right balance of hormones and to utilise them properly during each cycle will be seriously compromised. My opinion is that PMS is a multifaceted problem and that all the factors need to be looked at together.

Women are not a collection of separate parts. Everything in our bodies affects everything else. This fact is the real reason why over seventy years of research into PMS has drawn a blank – doctors and scientists have been approaching this condition in the wrong way. Rather than looking at women as a whole, with unique physical and emotional attributes and characteristics, they view the female body as something akin to a machine – a set of components. Research has been based around finding a faulty part, rather than looking at the interrelated systems and symptoms.

But women are not machines, and no one part is to blame. The relationship between the mind and the body has been well researched and documented, and factors affecting one will undoubtedly affect the other. It's valid to say that many of the symptoms of PMS are psychological, but if they had a purely psychological basis, they would be there throughout the month. And they are not.

What actually seems to be happening is that changes in the balance of female hormones – in other words, physical changes – are then giving rise to psychological changes. These psychological changes affect our wellbeing and our outlook. We may, for example, overeat or drink too much alcohol in order to cope. This affects the way we feel physically, and the way our bodies function, which, of course, has the potential to affect our emotions. It's a classic vicious circle.

It is much easier to make physical changes than it is to change our psychology. And because these two issues are interconnected, changes made on a physical level will impact on our emotional wellbeing. So the aim is not to look at all the different symptoms that we might be experiencing, and work on treating them separately. It's to achieve optimum health. This means looking at yourself as a whole person, making sure that you are eating well, correcting any vitamin and mineral deficiencies present, looking at your lifestyle in terms of stress, exercise and sleep, and then using certain herbs that have been shown to help with the symptoms of PMS, while encouraging your body to heal itself.

CHAPTER 5

The PMS Diet

What you eat is not only the foundation of your overall health. It's also an absolutely crucial factor in the elimination and prevention of PMS. In this chapter, I'll go through the basic elements of healthy eating, pointing out what foods are good for you and why, and which foods should be avoided.

If you think you've heard it all before, read it carefully — there are surprises in store. Take the time to follow the guidelines in this chapter; you will experience a revelation: not only a rapid relief from symptoms, but real results within the first month of changing the way you eat.

How can eating well really banish these monthly blues? First, let's look at some symptoms: irritability, aggressive outbursts, palpitations, forgetfulness, anxiety, confusion, inability to concentrate, crying spells, lack of sex drive, headaches/migraines and food cravings.

All symptoms of PMS, right? True — but they are also symptoms of something else. Every one of the symptoms listed above is a common feature of fluctuating blood sugar levels. In fact, it's this that is the key to eliminating PMS once and for all.

The 'little and often' approach to eating prevents blood sugar levels from dropping excessively, which in turn stops adrenaline from being released. When adrenaline is released, it blocks the uptake of the hormone progesterone in the second half of the menstrual cycle. So by the stabilising of blood sugar levels through healthy eating, the adrenaline is prevented from interfering with the progesterone, and symptoms are eliminated.

This theory presents a solution to the PMS problem that has been perplexing scientists for decades, and explains why women with PMS have the same sex hormone levels as women without. It's just that their bodies are not making use of them, because of low blood sugar levels.

Keeping blood sugar in balance

The link between blood sugar levels and adrenaline

After a meal, glucose produced by digestion is absorbed through the wall of the intestines into the bloodstream. At this point, there is, quite naturally, a high level of glucose in the blood. Your body takes what it immediately needs for energy and then produces insulin from the pancreas in an attempt to reduce the excess. Insulin transports glucose into the cells and the glucose that is not used for energy is changed into glycogen and stored in the liver and muscles to be used later. When glycogen levels are filled in the muscles and liver, the excess is stored as fat. It's this finely tuned system that usually keeps the glucose level in your blood at a healthy, well-balanced norm.

When the glucose level falls too low, adrenaline is released by the adrenal glands and glucagon is produced by the pancreas. Glucagon works in the opposite way from insulin, increasing blood glucose by encouraging the liver to turn some of its glycogen stores into glucose to give us quick energy. Adrenaline – a hormone normally released when we are under stress – enters the bloodstream because of a blood sugar imbalance.

In fact, research shows that women with PMS will experience more general stress in their lives than women without PMS.[1] I have found that when blood sugar is under control, women are much more able to cope with sources of stress in their lives such as work, relationships, money and parenting. The reason is that once blood sugar levels are stable, there are fewer surges of adrenaline, which add to feelings of stress. Levels of stress do not change – it's the way we perceive stressful situations that does.

Adrenaline and progesterone

Progesterone receptors, like oestrogen receptors, are found all over the body – in the breasts, womb, bone, liver, heart and brain. As we've seen, receptors work much like a lock, into which the 'key', in this case, hormones, fit. Each key has a different lock – in other words, every receptor uses a different hormone. So progesterone receptors will 'pick up' progesterone for the body to use.

But research has found that in the presence of adrenaline, these progesterone receptors are effectively blocked[2] and the body cannot utilise the progesterone, no matter how much of it there may be.

What makes your blood sugar rise and fall?

Blood sugar will automatically rise and fall during the day as you eat and drink. For most people in most situations, these fluctuations will all be within normal limits. However, different foods can cause your blood sugar to rise and fall outside them. The times you eat also have a dramatic effect on your blood sugar.

When you eat any food in its refined form, you digest it very quickly. Refined foods are no longer in their 'whole' state, and have been stripped of their natural goodness by various manufacturing processes. Two of the most widely used refined foods are sugar and white flour.

If digestion occurs too quickly, glucose enters the bloodstream too rapidly. This also happens when you eat any food or drink that has a stimulant effect, such as tea, coffee or chocolate. The initial stimulating 'high' quickly passes and you plummet down to a 'low' in which you feel tired and drained. So what do you need? Another stimulant, such as a cup of coffee or a bar of chocolate.

What's more, if you're in the habit of eating widely spaced meals, your blood glucose will drop to low levels during the gaps. The result? You'll feel the need for one of those quick boosts, such as a coffee. Meanwhile, your low glucose levels cause adrenaline to be released by the adrenal glands to encourage your liver to produce more glucose, to rectify the imbalance. You then have the opposite scenario – too much glucose in your blood, which means that your pancreas has to secrete more insulin in order to reduce your glucose levels. Your body is then on a roller-coaster ride of fluctuating blood sugar levels.

Studies show that women with PMS do not have different glucose levels from women without PMS, but they do eat more sugar, refined carbohydrates and dairy products.[3] It could be argued, then, that PMS causes women to crave sugar, cakes, and other 'instant boost' foods. But what if it's the other way round? What if eating sweets and biscuits causes changes in blood sugar levels, which then cause adrenaline to be released, which in turn interferes with the proper use of hormones (particularly progesterone), which then triggers PMS?

As we've seen, this is what happens: low blood sugar causes cravings, you satisfy them with a quick caffeine or carbohydrate fix, and blood sugar imbalances aren't far behind. So it's not the PMS that causes the cravings, it's out-of-kilter blood sugar levels – and these in turn exacerbate the symptoms of PMS.

Penny

Penny came to see me when she was fifty, saying that my book *Natural Alternatives to HRT* had 'saved' her. Nine years earlier she had developed PMS, which became very extreme: she would get very aggressive and be in tears for nearly a fortnight each month. She was a teacher in an infants' school, and was finding it difficult to function professionally in her job.

Penny was first prescribed a tranquilliser which she was not happy with, and then progesterone given as pessaries which she was asked to use six times a day every day of the month. She had been on this progesterone regime for eight years – and it had stopped her periods completely for the whole of that time – when in April 1998 she was doubled up with pain for 14 hours. Penny's doctor took her off the progesterone, and the pain stopped completely. The next month, Penny's period came back and she had been regular since. But after she stopped taking progesterone, she realised she had to do something else to stop premenstrual symptoms returning.

Penny read the dietary suggestions in my book and realised that she was a 'teapot' – a heavy tea drinker – so she changed to herbal teas. She added in agnus castus and also some supplements, including magnesium, which are recommended in the book. By the time she came to see me, she said her PMS was 'nothing at all' but that she was slightly irritable over the 24 hours before her period. She now wanted to make sure that she was not deficient in any nutrients and to prepare herself for the menopause. Her mineral analysis showed no deficiencies but high levels of copper from taking the hormone progesterone over eight years.

CHEW, CHEW, CHEW

A very simple tip to help curb your appetite, encourage weight loss and prevent cravings is to chew well. Take your time when eating. The first part of digestion starts in the mouth, so this helps you to digest and absorb your food better. But it also takes your brain twenty minutes to register you are full and have had enough to eat. If you eat more slowly, you will actually want to eat less.

Vital carbohydrates

To maintain a steady blood sugar level during the day, you should aim to eat complex carbohydrates – bread, pasta, cereals, potatoes and the like – as part of your main meals. Together with a little protein, and eaten little and often, complex carbohydrates can make an enormous difference to the way you feel throughout the day. In fact, sometimes just munching an oatcake between meals can be enough to keep cravings at bay.

If you wake during the night – at around 3 or 4 am – and cannot get back to sleep, it is very likely that your blood sugar level has dropped overnight and adrenaline has kicked in. Eating a small, starchy snack, such as half a slice of rye bread, one hour before going to bed will help you to sleep all the way through the night.

It's also important to ensure that the carbohydrates you eat are unrefined. In general terms, this means going for the 'whole' and 'brown' type rather than the 'white'. Wholewheat bread, brown rice and wholemeal flour are rich in essential vitamins, minerals, trace elements and valuable fibre, while their refined counterparts have been stripped of these elements. Some manufacturers now 'replace' lost nutrients by adding vitamins and minerals back into the final product, but these are still nutritionally inferior to the whole versions. They also lack fibre, which helps to slow down the digestive process and release a steady flow of energy.

And not only do carbohydrates keep your blood sugar in balance, but they help to increase blood serotonin levels, the 'calming' brain chemical that helps to lift mood and curb appetite. One study showed that simply changing your evening meal to one that is carbohydrate-rich and protein-poor for the second half of the cycle can reduce PMS symptoms, such as depression, tension, anger, confusion, sadness, fatigue, alertness and calmness.[4]

What to do about sugar

I would suggest that you eliminate sugar completely. Do not add it to any drinks or foods, such as tea, fruit or cereals, and avoid eating obviously sweet foods, such as chocolate. It's also important to read the labels, as sugar is added to many different foods, including tinned vegetables, soups, yoghurts, and even pasta sauces. A fruit yoghurt, for example, can contain up to eight teaspoons of sugar. A 'healthy' muesli bar can contain just as much.

Researchers have found that the higher the sugar content of a woman's diet, the more severe her premenstrual symptoms.[5] When we consider the fact that adrenaline is released when blood sugar levels fall – after a sugary snack, for example – and look at its blocking effect on progesterone, it's fairly clear that diet can have a dramatic effect on PMS symptoms.

Some researchers have called PMS a 'modern-day disease', not only because we have more periods than we used to (see pages 3–4), but also because of our 21st-century diet. On average, each of us consumes 2.25 pounds (1 kilogram) of sugar per week, and much of this is 'invisible' sugar, which is hidden in food that isn't strictly 'sweet'. In 1850, the world production of sugar was 1.5 million tons per year; that figure is now 75 million tons. We are eating 25 times the amount of sugar we ate 200 years ago.[6]

Sugar is just 'empty calories', and it provides no nutritional value. And in fact, sugar makes it more difficult for you to lose weight. Every time you eat, your body has a choice: it can burn that food as energy or it can store it as fat. Researchers have discovered that if more insulin is released, more of your food will be converted into fat. What's more, if food is actively being converted into fat, any previously stored fat fails to be broken down. So the more sugar you eat, the more insulin your body releases, and the more fat it stores.

We also know that the amount of sugar you consume can affect your immune system, and compromise your body's ability to fight any infections. It has been found that sugar detrimentally affects the process called phagocytosis, where white blood cells engulf and consume bacteria and foreign substances.[7] Sugar also encourages candida (see pages 154–9), which has been connected with premenstrual symptoms.

If sugar is out, what about artificial sweeteners? Leave these off the menu, too. Here's why.

Artificial sweeteners

If a food or drink is described as being 'low sugar', 'diet' or 'low calorie', it will usually contain a chemical sweetener such as aspartame. Unfortunately, aspartame has been linked to mood swings and depression because it alters the levels of the brain chemical serotonin.[8] Given that these are two of the prime emotional symptoms linked with PMS, it makes sense to avoid aspartame and any foods or drinks that contain it.

One of the classes of drugs used for PMS are SSRIs (selective serotonin re-uptake inhibitors), which are designed to optimise the use of serotonin. This helps to lift our mood and reduce appetite. Aspartame works in exactly the opposite way.

Women are often misled into believing that artificial sweeteners help to control weight. Ironically, however, it has been found that people who regularly use artificial sweeteners tend to gain weight because these sweeteners increase the appetite.[9] Aspartame is 180 times sweeter than sugar and it can lead to binge eating and weight problems.

There are other concerns about aspartame. In America, the Aspartame Toxicity Information Centre (www.holisticmed.com/aspartame) has been set up largely because of the concerns that aspartame may be causing more serious health problems.

When digested, aspartame releases methanol and two amino acids, aspartic acid and phenylalanine, into the body. Methanol converts to formaldehyde (formaldehyde, a toxin, is classed in the same group of substances as cyanide and arsenic) and then to formate or formic acid.[10] Amino acids are fundamental constituents of all proteins, and they also interact with each other. We normally ingest amino acids in proteins, taking them in in small quantities and in combination with other amino aids. Anyone eating aspartame, however, is ingesting aspartic acid and phenylalanine on their own, and in much larger quantities.

The result? Consuming aspartame can unbalance the metabolism of amino acids in the brain.[11] In other words, it affects the way our brains use amino acids. There are a variety of symptoms linked to regular consumption of aspartame. These include:

- Mood swings
- Memory loss
- Numbness and tingling
- Skin problems, such as urticaria and rashes
- Seizures and convulsions
- Headaches
- Eye problems
- Nausea and vomiting
- Depression.

There are also concerns that aspartame is addictive, and that people who drink three to four or more cans of diet soft drinks every day, or regularly chew sugar-free gum, may experience withdrawal symptoms as they try to stop.

My advice is to avoid any foods or drinks that contain artificial sweeteners. You will need to read the labels: they are found in everything from fizzy drinks, yoghurts, desserts and tinned foods to many convenience foods and much, much more.

As you give up sugar and artificial sweeteners, your taste buds will adapt. You'll begin to taste and appreciate the natural sweetness of foods such as parsnips and sweet potatoes. Sweetened, processed foods will begin to taste overly sweet. If you do find that you need a sweetener for some foods, try small amounts of honey, maple syrup, brown rice syrup or barley malt syrup. These are healthier alternatives because they not only have some nutritional value, but also are less likely to cause swings in your blood sugar levels.

FOOD-COMBINING AND PROTEIN-ONLY DIETS

I suggest that you eat little and often, basing your diet around good-quality complex carbohydrates, together with a small amount of healthy proteins such as pulses, fish and eggs. But there are quite a few other dietary suggestions around at the moment. Let's look at two that are grabbing a lot of the headlines.

You may have heard that it is better to follow a food-combining diet in order to lose weight. In this way of eating, protein and carbohydrates are consumed at separate meals, based on the belief that these two foods need different enzymes to be digested effectively. It is claimed that if they are eaten together, the undigested food is first stored in the intestines, where it ferments and causes bloating and flatulence. If this food is still not properly digested, and used as energy, it will be stored as fat. The theory behind this regime does not seem to have been proven scientifically, yet there are people who feel it has helped with digestive problems. But it can actually make things worse if you have PMS, as we'll see later on. Critics often say that food combining works as a weight-loss diet because it restricts food intake and helps people to become more aware of what they are eating.

Most traditional cultures do combine proteins and carbohydrates. The Japanese, for example, often have rice, fish and soya at a meal along with vegetables. So the problem lies not in eating carbohydrates per se, but in eating the wrong kind of them. Our modern-day diet tends to focus on refined carbohydrates, which are stripped of fibre and digested very quickly. Because of this, glucose enters the bloodstream too rapidly. The sharp, fast rise in blood glucose makes you feel momentarily good, but the 'high' quickly passes, plummeting you to a low point, at which adrenaline is released.

Glucose is the fastest-releasing carbohydrate because it needs no processing before it passes into the bloodstream, and it raises insulin levels very quickly. The Glycaemic Index was devised to

---

measure glucose levels in foods. In this index pure glucose is given a score of 100, and all foods are measured against this.

GLYCAEMIC INDEX (GI)

The GI essentially measures how quickly or slowly a food releases glucose into the bloodstream. The less refined a carbohydrate – for example, brown rice, whole grains and vegetables – the lower the GI. The fibre contained naturally in these foods slows down the

Sugars	GI Score	Fruit	GI Score
Glucose	100	Watermelon	72
Honey	87	Pineapple	66
Sucrose (sugar)	59	Melon	65
		Raisins	64
Grains and Cereals	*GI Score*	Banana	62
French baguette	95	Kiwi fruit	52
White rice	72	Grapes	46
Bagel	72	Orange juice	46
White bread	70	Orange	40
Ryvita	69	Apple juice	40
Brown rice	66	Apple	39
Muesli	66	Plum	39
Pastry	59	Pear	38
Basmati rice	58	Grapefruit	25
White spaghetti	50	Cherries	25
Porridge oats	49		
Instant noodles	46	*Vegetables*	*GI Score*
Wholegrain wheat bread	46	Parsnips (cooked)	97
Wholemeal spaghetti	42	Potatoes (baked)	85
Wholegrain rye bread	41	Potatoes (fried)	75
Barley	26	Potatoes (boiled)	70
		Beetroot (cooked)	64
Pulses	*GI Score*	Sweetcorn	59
Baked beans	48	Sweet potatoes	54
Butter beans	36	Potato crisps	54
Chickpeas	36	Peas	51
Blackeye beans	33	Carrots	49
Haricot beans	31		
Kidney beans	29		
Lentils	29		
Soya beans	15		

Glycaemic Index of common foods

release of sugars and gives them a lower GI. Similarly, whole fruit will have a lower GI than fruit juice, because fibre slows down the absorption of sugar.

The most important piece of information that has emerged from GI is that it is actually *beneficial* to combine proteins and carbohydrates. The presence of protein (either animal or vegetable) in food actually lowers its GI. So pulses such as lentils, which naturally contain both protein and carbohydrate, have a low GI.

The simplest way to work out the GI of a particular food without resorting to charts before every meal is to consider how refined it is. The more refined the food, the faster it will be digested, and the bigger its impact on your insulin levels. The result? If it's highly refined, it's going to make your PMS symptoms worse. Go for foods that are in their most natural state, and base your diet around fibre-rich foods such as brown rice. Once again, fibre slows down the release of sugars and gives them a lower GI.

For more information on the benefits of keeping your blood sugar in balance to lose weight, see my book *Natural Alternatives to Dieting*.

PROTEIN-ONLY DIETS

Diets that involved eating lots of protein, such as meat and eggs, but few carbohydrates, first became popular in the 1970s. Under this regime, even fruit intake is strictly limited because of its carbohydrate status. Recently the protein-only diet re-emerged and has now become the latest craze to sweep America, with a number of celebrities swearing by it as a way of losing weight fast.

The theory is that sweet and starchy foods make blood sugar levels rise sharply. And, as mentioned on page 52, when insulin levels are raised, more of your food is converted into fat, and you begin to put on weight. So it is believed that by cutting out anything that stops a surge of insulin, you will lose weight.

It sounds logical, and it can cause dramatic weight loss. However, in the long term, this type of diet is not only unhealthy – it can be dangerous. When the body is starved of carbohydrates it looks for energy in its glycogen stores. Because 4g (0.14oz) of water cling to every gram of glycogen, it is possible to lose a lot of weight very quickly. But the immediate weight loss is water, not fat. Only when the glycogen stores are depleted does the body start to dissolve fat.

A protein-only diet can cause an abnormal metabolic state called 'ketosis', because there is not enough carbohydrate stored in the liver for the body to use. Ketones accumulate in the blood, causing side-effects such as bad breath – a fruity odour of acetone – as well as poorer concentration, mood swings and bad memory. These are not symptoms that you will want to experience, especially when you could already be experiencing them in the run-up to your period. These same symptoms are experienced in cases of starvation, and in diabetes mellitus.

Added to this is the fact that a high-protein diet causes a build-up of nitrogen in the body. Nitrogen is a break-down product of protein, which is normally efficiently dealt with by the liver and kidneys and then excreted through the urine. When the protein content of the diet is very high, excess nitrogen builds up and can damage the liver and kidneys.

And if that's not enough, it is also known that the higher the amount of protein in your diet, the greater your risk of losing bone density (the extreme form of which is osteoporosis). Protein causes an acidic reaction in the body and calcium acts as a neutraliser. When you eat too much protein, your reserves of calcium, which are contained in your bones and teeth, are summoned to correct the imbalance. It is estimated that for every extra 15g (0.5oz) of protein you eat, 100g of calcium is lost in your urine.

Once again, my advice would be to avoid protein-only diets for two reasons. First and foremost, the body needs carbohydrates, and choosing the right kind – that is, complex whole carbohydrates – will undoubtedly encourage weight loss as well as help to reduce PMS problems by stabilising blood sugar levels. Secondly, the price of cutting out carbohydrates altogether is simply too high. In the long term, your overall health can be seriously damaged.

Caffeine

Caffeine has a diuretic effect on the body and so depletes valuable stores of vitamins and minerals that are essential for a healthy hormone balance. Caffeine is also a stimulant, whether it's found in tea, coffee, chocolate or caffeinated soft drinks, and as such it causes blood sugar levels to rise quickly, then swiftly drop. This contributes to the roller-coaster ride of blood sugar swings and the release of adrenaline. Avoid them whenever possible. Even better, cut them out of your diet completely and drink herbal teas and grain coffee, spring water and diluted pure fruit juices instead.

Tea contains tannin as well as caffeine. Tannin binds important minerals and prevents their absorption in the digestive tract. You may have an extremely nutritious diet, but if you drink tea at mealtimes, you can be excreting the majority of the minerals in your food without absorbing them.

If breast tenderness is your main premenstrual symptom, you should avoid any drinks or foods that contain caffeine. The active ingredients in caffeine are called methylxanthines and they have been proved to exacerbate breast pain, benign lumps and tenderness.[12] These methylxanthines are found in coffee, black tea, green tea, chocolate, cola and even decaffeinated coffee, as well as in medications that contain caffeine, such as some headache remedies.

Unfortunately, simply removing these substances in the second half of the cycle doesn't seem to work. They will have to be completely eliminated from your diet in order for you to see the benefits. Interestingly, just cutting down doesn't seem to have any effect at all. You need to go the whole way on this one. Some women can drink five cups of coffee a day and experience no breast problems premenstrually. Others can drink just one cup and find that cutting out that single cup of coffee will make a dramatic difference to breast symptoms. We are all unique, and it is really how sensitive you are to methylxanthines that makes the difference.

I would suggest that you eliminate caffeine gradually. Don't stop suddenly, overnight – you will suffer withdrawal symptoms, such as headaches, shaking and muscle cramps. It's much better to cut down slowly over a few weeks. Begin by substituting decaffeinated coffee for half of your total intake per day, then gradually change over to all decaffeinated. Then, slowly substitute other drinks, such as herbal teas and grain coffees. You will eventually have to eliminate decaffeinated coffee as well. Caffeine is one of three stimulants coffee contains, so even decaffeinated brands may have theobromine and theophylline in them, which will adversely affect your blood sugar levels. Quite apart from that, coffee is one of the most heavily sprayed plants in the world, and you will be ingesting high quantities of pesticides and other nasties with every cup. All of this will affect the overall function of your body and, ultimately, your PMS symptoms.

Fiona

Fiona was thirty-eight when she came to see me, complaining of excruciating breast tenderness in the second half of her cycle. She found it difficult to sleep because she couldn't get comfortable and didn't want her partner to touch her as it was so painful. She was a small, petite woman, and she felt that her breasts got so large premenstrually that they were out of all proportion to her size and she ended up feeling 'top heavy'. Fiona even had to wear a larger bra size in the second half of the cycle.

Fiona's health was good and she had no real problems other than this extreme breast tenderness and enlargement. We discussed her lifestyle and diet, and then she mentioned that she could drink up to ten cups of coffee a day. I talked about the relationship between coffee and breast discomfort, but initially she found it hard to believe that just one thing could be making all the difference. I suggested that she eliminate the coffee very gradually, as otherwise she could get terrible withdrawal symptoms such as headaches and shaking. She substituted half of her regular cups with decaffeinated coffee over the next week and gradually weaned herself off coffee over the next month. Eventually even the decaffeinated coffee had to go, as it contains the methylxanthines implicated in breast problems. It was, however, a good way to make the transition from ten cups of coffee a day to none.

She gradually substituted the coffee for grain coffees and herb teas and over the next three months the problem cleared up completely.

Eat oily foods

Does this seem an odd suggestion? Oil is traditionally associated with fat, and if you listen to the scare stories in the media, fat is something that should not pass our lips. In fact, most women follow, or have followed, a low- or no-fat diet for its health benefits, such as weight loss. But this pervading myth can do more damage than you'd think.

First and foremost, let me set the record straight. We all need fats. But it's the type that counts. Saturated fats are not good for us, and eating them can lead to a variety of health problems. However, some fats are not only important, they are essential for health − even more so for a woman with a health problem, particularly if it is hormone-related like PMS. These essential fats are, not surprisingly, known as 'essential fatty acids', or EFAs.

Do you suffer from any of these symptoms, alongside your normal pre-menstrual problems?

- Dry skin
- Cracked skin on heels or fingertips
- Hair falling out
- Lifeless hair
- Poor wound healing
- Dandruff
- Depression
- Irritability
- Soft or brittle nails
- Allergies
- Dry eyes
- Lack of motivation
- Aching joints
- Fatigue
- Difficulty losing weight
- High blood pressure
- Arthritis

These are all signs of an essential fatty acid deficiency. EFAs are found in foods such as nuts, seeds and oily fish. These essential fats are a vital component of every human cell and the body needs them to balance hormones, insulate nerve cells, and keep the skin and arteries supple and the body warm.

> **NOTE**
> Some of the symptoms associated with an EFA deficiency can also be caused by a thyroid imbalance, so it is worth seeing your doctor for a check-up (see also pages 159–62).

Hormone-like substances called prostaglandins are made from EFAs. Prostaglandins are present in most cells of the body and have been labelled with different letters and numbers – for example, PGE1, PGE2, PGF2. They influence smooth muscle contractions in the blood vessels, womb, intestines and much more. Certain prostaglandins, such as PGE2 and PGF2, have been linked to both period pains and endometriosis. (For more information on this subject, see my book *Nutritional Health Handbook for Women*.)

Prostaglandins

PGE1 is the prostaglandin most relevant to premenstrual symptoms. It has a balancing effect on blood sugar, which can help to prevent cravings for sweet foods and an increase in appetite, both of which are common with PMS. It helps to regulate the hormone prolactin, which is implicated in breast tenderness, and it reduces inflammation and prevents inappropriate blood clotting. PGE1 also helps to remove excess water because it has a beneficial effect on the kidneys. This is crucial, given that so many PMS symptoms are linked to water retention.

The essential fatty acid building block for PGE1 is linoleic acid, which is then converted to GLA (gamma-linolenic) and eventually to PGE1. Linoleic acid is found in polyunsaturated fats.

Polyunsaturated fats can be split into two types: omega 6 oils (which are found in unrefined safflower, corn, sesame and sunflower oils and also in the nuts and seeds themselves) and omega 3 oils (which are found in fish oils and linseed, or flaxseed, oil). The omega 6 oils contain linoleic acid, which is then converted into PGE1. Unfortunately, however, another type of prostaglandin called PGE2 can be produced from omega 6 oils. PGE2 can cause inflammation and inappropriate blood clotting, and is implicated in painful periods and endometriosis.

Overleaf is a diagram of how these 'good' and 'bad' prostaglandins are produced.

The best way to get to grips with how prostaglandins form is to imagine that omega 3 and omega 6 are two trains that run along a number of tracks. The omega 3 train needs to reach the PGE3 station, and the omega 6 train needs to reach the PGE1 station. If there are any obstacles on the omega 6 track, the train will be redirected towards the PGE2 station.

PGE3, which is produced from omega 3 oils, can also be classed as a 'good' prostaglandin because it helps to reduce inflammation and abnormal blood clotting. In the case of PMS, it is also important that good quantities of PGE1 are produced.

Foods that increase the production of 'bad' prostaglandins (PGE2)

As you can see from the chart on page 62, it is very important that you avoid all foods that are high in arachidonic acid (AA). Your body produces PGE2 from AA, the main sources of which are dairy products. This means

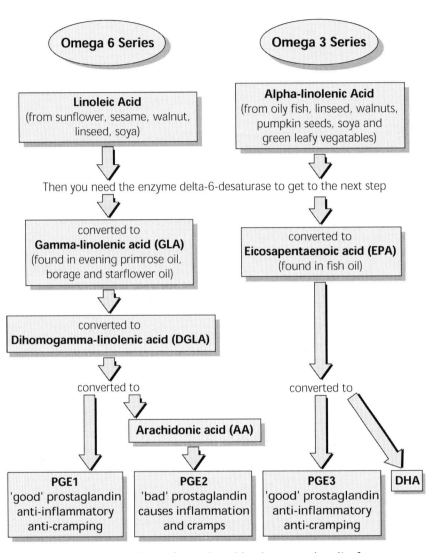

The production of good and bad prostaglandins]

eliminating or at least reducing dairy produce in any form, including milk, cheese, cottage cheese, yoghurt, butter and even dairy ice cream until your PMS symptoms are under control. These foods can then be reintroduced to your diet, but they must be eaten in moderation. AA is also present in red meat, but interestingly, although the saturated fat content of red meat is higher than in white meat, AA is higher in chicken and turkey than in red meat.

As a starting point, you will need to adjust your diet so that you eat more of those foods that begin the process of producing PGE1. You'll also need to reduce your intake of foods that cause your body to produce too many of the negative prostaglandins (PGE2). As well as providing your body with the right foods to kickstart the beneficial prostaglandin process, you also need to make sure that there is nothing in your diet or your lifestyle that will prevent your body from converting the right foods into healthy prostaglandins.

When working on the elimination of PMS symptoms, you'll need to eat foods rich in essential fats, but you should also take these fatty acids in supplement form. This will ensure that you get the correct balance, and that any deficiencies are corrected.

Factors that can block the conversion of essential fats

In order to start the ball rolling, your body needs to convert the omega 6 series, linoleic acid (LA), into gamma-linolenic acid (GLA). It has been discovered that many women with PMS have an inherent problem that makes converting essential fatty acids to GLA difficult.[13]

If you have this problem and are also a big dairy food eater, you will undoubtedly end up with very little PGE1 and too much PGE2. Obviously, when the balance is tipped in that direction, you'll be much more likely to suffer PMS symptoms and possibly even period pains or cramps.

There are a number of other factors that can hamper the conversion of linoleic acid to GLA. These include stress, a diet high in sugar, saturated fats and margarines, and deficiencies of vitamin B6, magnesium and zinc. An enzyme called delta–6–desaturase helps your body make this conversion (see chart opposite) and this enzyme needs B6, magnesium and zinc to do its job.

Monounsaturated fats (omega 9) are not classed as essential fatty acids, but they can boost your health. Olive oil, for example, is high in monounsaturated fats, which are believed to lower the risk of heart attack and other circulatory problems. Use olive oil or butter for cooking and frying as they are more stable when heated than polyunsaturated oils (found in vegetable oils). Whenever possible, use cooking techniques other than frying, such as baking, steaming, roasting and grilling.

Oils can easily become damaged, so it's essential that you take care when choosing, storing and using them. If oils are heated over too high a flame, left in sunlight or reused after cooking, they can lose their beneficial effects.

Buy cold-pressed, unrefined vegetable oils or extra-virgin olive oil. A number of supermarkets now sell organic oils, which are better still because no chemicals will have been used in their production. Unfortunately, standard supermarket oils are manufactured and extracted using chemicals and heat. This destroys the quality of the oil and the nutritional content. Store your oil away from sunlight and do not be tempted to reuse it after cooking.

> **MARGARINE VERSUS BUTTER**
>
> Hydrogenated vegetable oil is listed in the ingredients of most margarines and also many fast foods, crisps, biscuits and crackers. The process of hydrogenation (which basically makes a fat more solid and spreadable) changes the essential unsaturated fats contained in the food into trans fatty acids, which have been linked to all sorts of problems, including an increased risk of heart attack and an inability to absorb essential fats.[14]
>
> For this reason, I would recommend using butter, particularly the organic kind now stocked by most supermarkets, or unhydrogenated margarine, which you can get from health food shops, rather than ordinary margarine. Although margarine is manufactured from polyunsaturated fats, these 'good' fats become 'trans fats' in the hydrogenation process. Trans fats have a plasticky quality that makes them hard to eliminate from your body. They also make it more difficult for your body to produce the 'good' prostaglandins from the food you eat. Why put your body under extra pressure to deal with a substance that you do not really need to eat?

Saturated fats

Saturated fats are not essential for your health – in fact, this is one type of fat you could do without. These fats come mainly from animals, and are contained in foods such as meat, eggs and dairy products. They are also present in tropical oils like palm and coconut. Saturated fats can be detrimental to your health, especially when consumed in large amounts.

For one thing, saturated fats can contribute to weight gain. The more saturated a fat becomes, the harder it is to digest, so it is deposited in the body. Butter, coconut oil and palm oil are the saturated fats most easily assimilated by the body, so they are less harmful. Fat from beef, lamb and pork are the most difficult to digest because they are hard at body temperature.

Saturated fats can also block other nutrients. They interfere with your body's absorption of essential fatty acids that you need to eliminate PMS.

The saturated fats in red meat and poultry produce hormones called prostaglandins. And these are not the healthy prostaglandins that can be created by essential fatty acids (see page 61), which are important for alleviating premenstrual symptoms.

Alcohol

While you are changing your diet in order to get PMS under control, it's vital to keep your drinking at sensible levels, or cut it out completely. A couple of units (2 glasses of wine) a week is the maximum you should drink while you are concentrating on conquering PMS. Why is this? First of all, it's important that you give your liver a rest so that it can do its job of detoxifying and excreting your hormones efficiently. Secondly, alcohol can cause blood sugar fluctuations, which need to be controlled if PMS is to be treated successfully. Alcohol is basically a liquid carbohydrate that enters the bloodstream fairly rapidly, and of course has no fibre to slow it down. As it goes into the bloodstream, it boosts the secretion of insulin, which subsequently causes a drop in blood sugar.

Alcohol takes its toll on your liver (see pages 76–7), and can compromise that organ's ability to detoxify your system efficiently, which is one of its main roles. It contributes to blood sugar imbalances and acts as an antinutrient, which means that it blocks out the nutritional value of food by depleting vitamins and minerals. Alcohol can interfere with the metabolism of essential fatty acids, which as we've seen are absolutely crucial if you're to control PMS. Alcohol is also full of empty calories – just one glass of wine contains about 100 calories, while a pint of beer provides a whopping 200.

You may be wondering how all this fits in with the idea that red wine is good for us. Most of us have heard of the French paradox. The French eat possibly even more saturated fat, for example in meat and cheese, than we do in Britain, and yet their heart disease rate is substantially lower. The reason for this apparent anomaly is that grapes contain an antioxidant called resveratrol, which decreases the 'stickiness' of the blood platelets and prevents the blood vessels from narrowing. Resveratrol is mainly contained in the skin of grapes, which is why red wine seems to be more effective than white. Red wine is made from whole grapes, including the skin and pips, whereas white wine is made from only the flesh of the grape. Scientists have compared the effect of alcoholic and non-alcoholic red wines and found that the non-alcoholic version is actually better for the heart.[15]

Once you have eliminated your premenstrual symptoms, the best approach is to drink alcohol in moderation and save it mainly for the weekend or special occasions. Do not drink every night and, when you do, don't have more than two glasses of wine or beer at a time.

Phytoestrogens

Phytoestrogens are literally plant oestrogens – in other words, plants that have an oestrogenic effect. It may sound odd to suggest using supplemental oestrogen, even in a natural form, given that one prevailing theory is that PMS is caused by too much oestrogen. Surely on this basis, extra oestrogen would make the situation worse?

But these phytoestrogens have a very interesting effect on the body. They can increase oestrogen levels when they are low and reduce them when are too high.[16] This seems to explain why phytoestrogens can reduce hot flushes in menopausal women (which are thought to be due to a lack of oestrogen), but also reduce the incidence of breast cancer (which can be due to a problem with oestrogen).

These phytoestrogens have a balancing effect on oestrogen regardless of whether it is too high or too low, so it is an ideal form of treatment for PMS. Because researchers simply cannot agree on whether PMS is caused by high levels of oestrogen and inadequate progesterone, or inadequate oestrogen, or a combination of the two, it's clear that a treatment designed to address all of these issues is not only useful but essential.

When you give your body the right tools – in this case, food – it will balance itself. You don't even have to know where the imbalance lies. The fact that you feel unwell for a week or so leading up to your period is evidence that there is a fundamental imbalance.

Phytoestrogens are found in almost all fruit, vegetables and cereals, but they are most beneficial in the form of isoflavones, which are found in legumes or pulses such as soya, lentils, chickpeas and so on. Beans are easy to cook and are delicious when added to salads, soups and casseroles. Most beans (although not lentils) need to be soaked, sometimes overnight, before cooking. Alternatively, you can buy organic beans in tins from most supermarkets. Hummus is made from chickpeas, and it is available ready-made from most supermarkets.

Another interesting aspect of phytoestrogens is that they help to stimulate the production of SHBG (sex hormone-binding globulin).[17] SHBG is a protein produced by the liver that binds sex hormones, such as oestrogen and testosterone, in order to control how much is circulating in the blood at any one time. If you have the correct amount of SHBG, there will be a balancing effect on your hormones, ensuring that just the right amount is present in your body.

The concept of using SHBG on PMS was tested in a study published in 2000. A group of women were asked to follow a low-fat vegetarian diet. Researchers found that for these women, SHBG levels went up and PMS symptoms were significantly reduced while they were on the diet. The women experienced fewer mood swings and less water retention. What's more, the increased SHBG levels led to a reduction in both the intensity and the duration of period pains.[18]

Interestingly, this low-fat vegetarian diet – which consisted of grains, vegetables, legumes and fruit – more closely resembles a traditional way of eating than our 21st-century diet. And cutting out cheese and other dairy produce, which is high in fat, means that the 'bad' prostaglandins are not produced, which are, of course, one of the main causes of period pains and other hormone-related problems.

Because these phytoestrogens have a balancing effect on your hormones, it is important to include them in your diet. Research has also shown that phytoestrogens can help to produce lighter periods, and to lengthen the cycle in women whose cycles are too short.[19] So not only will they help to eliminate PMS symptoms, but they can help to provide more comfortable periods as well.

Phytoestrogens also have other positive benefits. Soya beans have been found to contain at least five compounds believed to inhibit cancer. Most of the research in this area has focused on breast cancer, mainly because Japanese women have only one-sixth the rate of breast cancer that Western women have. It appears that when Japanese women move to the West, their rate rises to that of Western women.[20] The majority of Asian women do not experience premenstrual breast discomfort, either.

These phytoestrogens appear to fit into oestrogen receptors on breast cells. Although they are a source of oestrogen, they are probably too weak to stimulate the cells to produce cancer. What seems to happen is that these weak oestrogens *block* the oestrogen receptors and prevent cancer from developing.

As well as benefiting the hormones, phytoestrogens also have a positive effect on your cardiovascular health. Studies have shown that soya can lower the level of cholesterol, particularly the 'bad' cholesterol (LDL).[21]

LINSEEDS

Flaxseeds, also known as linseeds, contain both essential fatty acids (EFAs omega 3 and omega 6), which are extremely important in combating PMS (see page 61). They also contain phytoestrogens (naturally occurring oestrogens found in plants), so they are an important food to include in your daily diet. Research has shown that giving women 10g of ground linseeds per day increases the regularity of the cycle and improves ovulation.[22] You can also take linseed oil in supplement form (see page 141).

Variety is the key to a healthy diet. Phytoestrogens are also found in garlic, celery, seeds (including linseeds, as seen in the box, sesame seeds and sunflower seeds), grains such as rice and oats, certain fruits, vegetables, alfalfa and mung beansprouts, and herbs such as sage, fennel and parsley. For further information on the different types of phytoestrogens (isoflavones, lignans and coumestans) and how to eat a healthy diet cooking with these foods, see my book *Natural Alternatives to HRT Cookbook*.

Genetically modified foods

This is the ultimate can of worms, and I've discussed it in some detail in my book *Natural Alternatives to HRT*. Genetic modification involves tampering with the DNA of a plant or animal. Even patent advocates of the process have to admit that it bypasses the natural evolutionary process, and we do not know yet what the price of that may be. For that reason, I suggest that everyone avoids buying, eating or using genetically modified products. Stick to organic: organic foods and other products are not genetically modified.

Salt

In general, most of us eat too much salt, which increases the potential for water retention. In Chapter 10 I look at the various recommendations for eliminating this problem, but it's undoubtedly key to monitor the amount of salt you are eating, and make changes where necessary.

The trouble is that salt is 'hidden' in a wide range of foods, and particularly those marketed to people who are trying to lose weight: where the fat content is reduced, more salt is often added to keep the food tasty. A high salt intake could mean that we can be carrying around an extra 1.8kg (4lb) in weight due to water retention.

The World Health Organization recommends that we do not eat more than 6g (1 rounded teaspoon) of salt per day. But most people end up eating about 9g a salt a day – it is easy to consume too much without realising it. One burger in a bun can contain 6g, two slices of wholemeal bread 1.2g and a slice of cheese and tomato pizza 5.3g. Two slices of bread contain more salt than a packet of crisps.

Tips for reducing salt intake

- Only use salt in cooking; do not add it to your food at the table. Some people have a habit of sprinkling salt on their food without even tasting it first.
- To help reduce your intake of salt, use other flavourings such as herbs, garlic or lemon, try a low-salt product or use tamari (wheat-free) soya sauce in moderation.
- Read the labels. Many tinned and processed foods have a high salt content, including some surprise items such as vegetables. If you are buying tinned tuna, for example, choose brands packed in sunflower oil or spring water rather than brine. If you buy tinned beans in salt water, make sure you drain off the liquid. It is better to avoid processed foods altogether so that you can control how much salt is added.

Dairy foods

Dairy foods are, unfortunately, not advised for women with PMS. There are several problems associated with cheese, milk, butter and yoghurt. First and foremost, most dairy foods are high in saturated fat (see pages 64–5), which can lead to a variety of different problems. Secondly, however, dairy produce can interfere with your body's ability to produce the 'good' prostaglandins (see page 61–2) that are so crucial for controlling PMS, and particularly breast tenderness.

Too much dairy food can also block the absorption of magnesium, a vital mineral where PMS is concerned. You might remember that some studies of women with PMS show they have lower levels of magnesium. Ultimately, you need to avoid anything that makes the uptake of a vital mineral more difficult. Magnesium is especially important when your symptoms are predominantly linked to anxiety, tension and mood swings.

You may be concerned about your calcium intake if you are avoiding dairy produce. Don't worry. There are many other foods that contain high levels of calcium, including sesame seeds, leafy green vegetables, nuts (especially brazil nuts and almonds), fish (particularly tinned salmon, as it includes the bones), watercress, figs, broccoli and seaweed. And by adding a good multivitamin and mineral (see page 108) to your daily diet, you will ensure not only that you are getting 'insurance' levels of this key mineral, but also that you will be getting other important vitamins and minerals that help your body to function better.

So keep your dairy intake to a minimum. Any dairy produce that you do eat should be organic, which is free of the harmful effects of antibiotics and other chemicals, many of which can exacerbate health problems. The best dairy product is yoghurt. When it contains a live culture, such as lactobacillus acidophilus or bifidus, it can be enormously beneficial. These 'healthy' bacteria are natural inhabitants of the gut, and they form one of the key defences of the immune system, keeping unhealthy bacteria and invaders, such as yeast infections and viruses, at bay. 'Live' yoghurts normally contain cultures, but the cartons can be marked in a variety of different ways. 'Bio', for example, usually means 'live' and will contain a culture like lactobacillus. When yoghurts are heat-treated, they lose their original culture, so you will not experience any health benefits from eating them. Similarly, heavily flavoured fruit yoghurts and those with a high sugar content can be low in or devoid of healthy bacteria. Wherever possible, go for plain, organic, live yoghurts and add a little fresh fruit and perhaps honey to flavour them.

Avoid drinks that claim to contain 'friendly bacteria'. Some brands are better than others, but those that contain sugar should be off the menu. If you drink them you will simply exacerbate any blood sugar problems rather than fulfil the aim of adding healthy bacteria to your diet.

Your healthy eating plan

The aim of this eating plan is to keep your blood sugar in balance, to ensure that you are getting enough essential fatty acids, to provide a good supply of phytoestrogens and to include all those foods that are known to encourage health and wellbeing.

As well as making sure that you are eating well, you also should ensure that you eat little and often. Do not go more than three hours without food and if you start to feel lightheaded or dizzy sooner, don't hesitate to eat.

Eating well to balance your blood sugar isn't difficult. In fact, it requires very little more than upgrading your carbohydrates to their more natural, whole form, and watching when you eat.

BLOOD SUGAR CHECKLIST

Answer the following questions:

1 Are you rarely wide awake within twenty minutes of rising?
2 Do you need tea, coffee or a cigarette to get you going in the morning?
3 Do you really like sweet foods?
4 Do you crave bread, cereal, popcorn or pasta?
5 Do you feel you 'need' an alcoholic drink on most days?
6 Are you overweight and unable to shift the extra kilos?
7 Do you often have energy slumps during the day or after meals?
8 Do you often have mood swings or difficulty concentrating?
9 Do you get dizzy or irritable if you go six hours without food?
10 Do you often find you overreact to stress?
11 Do you often get irritable, angry or aggressive unexpectedly?
12 Is your energy level lower now than it used to be?
13 Do you ever lie about how much sweet food you have eaten?
14 Do you ever keep a supply of sweet food close to hand?
15 Do you feel you could never give up bread?

If you answered 'Yes' to eight or more of the questions above, then it is very likely that your blood sugar is fluctuating quite markedly during the day, making you more prone to PMS symptoms.
(The above questions are reproduced with the kind permission of Patrick Holford, author of *The 30 Day Fat Burner Diet*.)

Top tips for healthy eating

- Eat unrefined complex carbohydrates including wholewheat bread, potatoes, brown rice, millet, oats, rye, and so on.
- Dilute pure fruit juice. A glass of orange juice could contain the juice of up to eight oranges. Obviously you could not physically eat eight oranges at one time! Pure fruit juice is very concentrated and will not contain any of the natural fibre content of the fruit itself. For this reason, it will have a dramatic effect on your blood sugar. While it's certainly healthier and less severe than the effect of ordinary sugar, it is still better to dilute fruit juice, and to drink more apple than orange juice. And vary your juice intake. Choosing lots of different juices will ensure that you are getting a good range of vital nutrients.
- Eat breakfast, even if it's something small. Porridge oats are a healthy choice, not only because they are a good form of complex carbohydrates, but also because they are rich in B vitamins, which protect the health of your nervous system.
- Eat small frequent meals, no more than three hours apart.
- Reduce, and preferably avoid, all stimulants, including tea, coffee, chocolate, nicotine and canned drinks that contain caffeine.
- Don't eat refined carbohydrates. Avoid 'white' in general. Remember that white flour is in many things, such as cakes, biscuits, pastries and white bread.
- Don't eat sugar or sugary foods, including chocolate, sweets, biscuits, pastries and soft drinks.
- Eat less dried fruit. This is important because when a fruit is dried, the water is removed, and the fruit sugar becomes more concentrated. So the effect on blood sugar is more extreme. You could try mixing in nuts with dried fruit, which will slow down the reaction by adding protein.
- Try to eat at least five portions of fruit and vegetables a day.
- When eating animal protein such as fish, only eat as much as will fit into the palm of one hand at any one meal.

Shopping list

Think about including the foods listed below on your shopping list and leaving out anything with sugar, caffeine, artificial sweeteners, preservatives or additives, and convenience foods in general.

Buy organic where possible. If your budget is limited and you are unsure of what to prioritise in terms of organic produce, go for organic grains, as in porridge, brown rice and wholemeal bread. Even if this is the only organic part of your diet it can make a huge difference. Grains are very small, so they can absorb more pesticides than other foods.

Remember that organic produce, such as carrots and potatoes, does not need to be peeled. Most of the nutrients of vegetables and fruits are concentrated just under the skin. Just wash and scrub them carefully and prepare as normal.

- Plenty of fresh vegetables and fruit
- Whole brown rice, oats, millet, etc.
- Wholewheat pasta
- Wholemeal flour
- Wholemeal bread, rye bread, crackers
- Beans such as lentils, aduki beans, chickpeas, kidney beans, etc.
- Sea salt or rock salt (commercial table salt has chemicals added to it to make it flow freely)
- Nuts and seeds
- Fish
- Organic dairy produce in moderation, including live plain yoghurt
- Free-range, organic eggs
- Dried fruit in moderation (for example, raisins, apricots, dates, sultanas, and so on)
- Butter and/or unhydrogenated margarine
- Cold-pressed unrefined vegetable oils, such as sesame and sunflower oils for dressings (choose extra-virgin olive oil for light cooking)
- Coffee substitutes, such as grain coffees
- Tea alternatives, such as herb teas, fruit teas, green tea (in moderation, as it contains a small amount of caffeine), Rooibosch (caffeine-free South African tea)
- Unsweetened pure fruit juices, diluted. Avoid flavoured mineral waters, squash and soft drinks.
- A little honey, maple syrup, barley malt or concentrated apple juice for sweetening

If you would like to know some interesting ways to cook with these natural ingredients, see my book *Natural Alternatives to HRT Cookbook*.

CHAPTER 6

Lifestyle Changes

Changing your diet will have a dramatic effect on the way you look and feel, and is the single most important key to controlling and curing PMS. But there are also a number of other factors that affect the way your body works and responds to external stimuli that can exacerbate PMS in susceptible women.

We know, for example, that exercise is an extremely important part of a healthy lifestyle, but you may be unaware that it also affects PMS symptoms. It's the same with sleep, and a number of other factors. Adopting healthy habits in all areas of our lives can ensure not only that we reach and maintain optimum health, but that our bodies work effectively and efficiently to meet the demands of modern-day living. There is no better way to address PMS once and for all than by making changes towards wellbeing.

It's now generally known that your body's hormonal and more general physical balance is directly affected by forces in the environment. In particular, you need to watch out for a group of foreign oestrogens known as 'xenoestrogens'.

Xenoestrogens

When you are helping restore your own physical health and working on eliminating PMS, you need to make sure that there are no hormones coming in from outside that could upset your state of balance. Unfortunately, this is increasingly difficult: we are now exposed to forms of oestrogen in the environment.

Xenoestrogens are oestrogen-like chemicals present in some pesticides or plastics. These 'foreign oestrogens' are having a dramatic effect on wildlife. For example, some fish are growing both male and female sex organs, and male alligators are becoming feminised, with hormonal levels altered to such an extent that reproduction is difficult. There's no doubt that all of us are affected by xenoestrogens, and they may be at the root of many of our female hormone problems, including PMS.

Xenoestrogens are stored in body fat and can affect men and women differently. Overweight people tend to have higher concentrations because xenoestrogens are lipophilic – meaning that they love fat.

Increasing levels of xenoestrogens in our environment have coincided with an earlier onset of puberty in girls, as I mentioned earlier in this book. At the turn of the century the average age for puberty to begin was fifteen. Now girls as young as eight are growing breasts and pubic hair. It has been found that girls can enter puberty almost a year earlier if their pregnant mothers had higher levels of two synthetic chemicals, PCBs and DDT, while they were pregnant.[1]

An earlier onset of puberty will increase the number of cycles a woman has in her lifetime – and increase the possibility of developing PMS.

How do you avoid xenoestrogens? Here are a number of ways to do it.

- There are 3,900 brands of insecticide, herbicide and fungicide that are approved for use in Britain, and some fruits and vegetables are sprayed as many as ten times before they reach the supermarket shelves. What's the answer? Buy as much organic as you can afford.
- Avoid, as far as possible, food and drinks in plastic containers or wrapped in plastic. Don't store any fatty foods such as cheese or meat in plastic wrap. Because xenoestrogens are lipophilic, or fat-loving, they will tend to migrate into foods with a high fat content. Remove food from plastic packaging as soon as possible.
- Reduce your intake of saturated fats. There are two reasons for this. First of all, by eating them you lay down fat stores that present a welcome home for xenoestrogens. Secondly, the fat you take in is likely to contain xenoestrogens from the animal's environment.
- Do not heat food in plastic, especially in a microwave oven.
- Increase your intake of fibre (see pages 55–6), which helps to prevent the absorption of oestrogenic chemicals into your bloodstream.
- Eat more cruciferous vegetables, such as broccoli, Brussels sprouts, cabbage and cauliflower. These are high in a substance call indole-3-carbinol, which helps to prevent toxic oestrogen from being absorbed in your body, while at the same time encouraging its elimination.

- Eat phytoestrogens (see pages 66–8) such as soya, chickpeas and lentils, which can reduce the toxic forms of oestrogen in your body.
- Buy 'natural' cleaning products for your home, to reduce the number of potentially xenoestrogenic chemicals in your household.
- Use natural toiletries – this is particularly important for anything that is rubbed into your skin.

Smoking

You may be wondering why I'm bringing smoking into a discussion on PMS. Certainly the problems associated with smoking are well known. They include an increased risk of lung cancer and emphysema, and damage to the developing baby during pregnancy.

But what you probably don't know is that smoking has an extremely negative effect on your hormones: it reduces your oestrogen levels. Smoking has been linked with infertility in women[2] and can bring on an early menopause because it brings down oestrogen levels to those more often seen in a menopausal woman.[3]

Sadly, there's more. Tobacco contains more than 4,000 compounds, including carbon monoxide, oxide of nitrogen, ammonia, aromatic hydrocarbons, hydrogen cyanide, vinyl chloride, nicotine, lead and cadmium.

When I do a mineral test on women who smoke (see pages 167–9), they tend to have high levels of a heavy toxic metal called cadmium. Cadmium can stop the utilisation of zinc, a mineral that is especially important for the health of the reproductive system. Once you stop smoking, it's a good idea to take antioxidants such as vitamin C to help your body eliminate accumulated cadmium.

When you are trying to keep your hormone levels in balance, it is extremely important that you eliminate anything, such as smoking, that will upset that delicate balance. If you need help to give up, acupuncture and hypnotherapy can be useful. I would suggest you try to avoid nicotine patches and gums, as you can actually become addicted to them.

> **YOUR LIVER**
> The liver, the largest gland in your body, is in effect your waste disposal unit – not only for toxins, waste products, drugs and alcohol, but also for hormones. If your liver is not functioning

efficiently, old hormones can accumulate after each menstrual cycle. And unless they are deactivated by the liver, they can return to the bloodstream and cause hormonal imbalances.

The liver deals with oestrogen so it can be eliminated safely from the body. As discussed on page 28, oestrogen is not one hormone, but a group of hormones, and includes oestradiol, oestrone and oestriol. Oestrogen is secreted by the ovaries in the form of oestradiol and the liver metabolises oestradiol to oestrone and oestriol. The liver's ability to efficiently convert oestradiol, the most carcinogenic oestrogen, to oestriol is very important because oestriol is the safest and least active form of oestrogen.

The liver also performs other functions that have a bearing not only on your premenstrual symptoms but also on your general health. Among its many tasks are the storage and filtration of blood, the secretion of bile, and numerous metabolic functions, including the conversion of sugars into glycogen, the form in which carbohydrates are stored in your body. It plays a vital part in metabolising fat so that it is broken down properly, and it helps to use up fat to produce energy. The liver also help to optimise thyroid function.

KEEPING YOUR LIVER HEALTHY

As well as avoiding substances that can compromise your liver function, such as alcohol, saturated fats and refined sugar, you can also take substances to help liver function. The B vitamins are especially important because they are essential if the liver is to be able to convert oestradiol into the harmless oestriol.

Milk thistle (*Silybum marianum*) is an excellent herb for the liver. A number of studies have shown that it can boost the number of new liver cells to replace old damaged ones.[4] Dandelion (*Taraxacum officinale*) is useful, too, as it helps to improve liver function and can help with general detoxification and elimination of hormones.

A good multivitamin and mineral (see page 108) is essential for making sure that you have all the nutrients – for example, zinc, calcium and B vitamins – that your liver needs in order to operate efficiently. The antioxidant vitamins, such as vitamin C, vitamin E and beta-carotene, are also important, and vitamin C should be taken in addition to the multivitamin and mineral to ensure that you have adequate levels in your blood.

Stress

Stress undoubtedly lies at the root of many modern-day health conditions, so not surprisingly it is also often implicated in PMS. As discussed on page 48, adrenaline is released by the adrenal gland when blood sugar drops. It is also released during the 'fight or flight' mechanism, when we are stressed. This has a dramatic effect on the female hormone system, and our bodies are unable to use progesterone properly in the second half the cycle when adrenaline is present. The result? Premenstrual symptoms.

Our modern lifestyles contain many different stressful situations – traffic jams, late trains, missed appointments, financial worries, work, family responsibilities, and simply day-to-day living at a top-speed pace. Adrenaline is released almost constantly when we are stressed, and its effect can be very powerful. The heart speeds up and the arteries tighten to raise blood pressure. Our livers immediately release emergency stores of glucose into the bloodstream to give us instant energy to fight or run. And digestion shuts down, because the energy necessary for digestion must be diverted elsewhere. The clotting ability of our blood is also increased, in the event of a potential injury.

In prehistoric times, this adrenaline response was necessary for an immediate reaction to a dangerous situation. However, once the threat diminished, adrenaline levels would return to normal, all in a short space of time.

The problem with our modern lifestyle is that perceived threats are almost continuous, which means that adrenaline is constantly released and is continuously affecting us physically. We may, for instance, sit in traffic jams, becoming more and more stressed, while trying to eat our lunch. And we will sit there and seethe, unable to take action such as running or fighting, as we would have done in response to a dangerous situation in the past. Furthermore, these periods in which adrenaline is surging through our bodies are prolonged – sometimes for hours on end. So we may try to eat lunch when our digestion has shut down, and, more dangerously, our risk of strokes and heart attacks increases dramatically, as the time it takes to clot our blood is increased. Because we aren't getting the energy we need from our food, our blood sugar drops, which means that we could literally be 'running on adrenaline', causing us to become more and more stressed and unable to cope.

It is interesting that women with PMS are known to see daily stressors as more stressful premenstrually and less stressful postmenstrually than similar events experienced by women without PMS – and what's more, women with PMS tend to experience more general stress in their lives than women without PMS.[5] This could be due to the effects of all this cumulative adrenaline surging round the body.

Stress can directly affect your reproductive system. Women going through a bereavement or other kind of trauma, for instance, can stop having periods.[6] The hormone prolactin can also be released when you are under stress, and this is known to aggravate breast tenderness and may also be connected with depression. In this connection it's interesting to note that the herb St John's wort (*Hypericum perforatum*), although well documented for its effects on depression (see pages 115–16), has been found to help lower prolactin levels.[7]

Your immune system can also be compromised if you are under stress. You will then be more prone to infections and also find it difficult to fight them off when you do succumb. In some instances, infections can linger on for weeks.

The adrenals and stress

The adrenal glands are responsible for pumping out all that adrenaline in response to stress, or when blood sugar levels are low. But these glands do much more than this. The adrenal glands sit on top of the kidneys and are made up of two parts, the medulla and the cortex. It is the medulla that produces adrenaline, while the cortex, which is stimulated by hormones from the pituitary gland, produces three kinds of hormones that are absolutely crucial for controlling premenstrual symptoms: cortisol, aldosterone, and the sex hormones oestrogen and testosterone.

Cortisol helps to control fat, protein and carbohydrate metabolism. In turn, it helps energy production, thyroid hormone production and the strength of our immune systems. Cortisol is produced at different levels during the day. This rhythm is as important as the amount of cortisol that your adrenals are producing. Cortisol should be highest in the morning and lowest at night – a logical rhythm, in that it is highest when you are ready for the day ahead and lowest when you are going to bed.

When you are under stress, the normal rhythm of your stress hormones can be upset. Levels of cortisol, in particular, can be disturbed. This can then affect the body in many ways. Low energy levels can, for example, be due to an abnormal adrenal rhythm, particularly if you find it difficult to get up in the morning.

We are more prone to osteoporosis if the adrenal glands are overworking, because excessively high levels of cortisol will prevent the proper build-up of bone. And as we've seen, the reproductive system is especially susceptible to stress, which can cause your periods to stop or become irregular, or cause the symptoms of PMS. Your immune system and thyroid function (see pages 159–62) can also be compromised if the adrenal glands are not doing their job properly.

STRESS INDEX

It is now possible to look at your stress levels by measuring the secretion of hormones from the adrenal glands. This test measures the rhythm of the adrenal glands by using four saliva samples over a day, which are collected at home and then sent to the lab for analysis. If you would like to know more about this test, please contact me (see page 187).

Your adrenals also produce a hormone called aldosterone, which acts on the kidneys to regulate salt and water balance. So the healthy production of this hormone is crucial for eliminating premenstrual symptoms associated with water retention and bloating.

If you have been under continual stress or your blood sugar levels have been fluctuating owing to skipped meals and/or a high intake of caffeine or sugar, your adrenals can become 'exhausted'. They will not function properly, and their ability to produce cortisol and aldosterone in normal amounts will be compromised. The result can be continual feelings of stress and exhaustion, including lethargy, and a tendency to succumb to repeated minor illnesses and infection. Finally, 'worn-out' adrenal glands can lead to increased frequency and severity of premenstrual symptoms – only one reason why it's essential that you keep them healthy.

There are other problems connected with the adrenal glands. These glands produce sex hormones (oestrogen and testosterone) in addition to those produced by the ovaries. If they are overstimulated, they can secrete too much of the male hormones. This will stop ovulation, and when ovulation ceases, the ovaries begin to secrete even more testosterone. So you end up with large hormonal imbalances.

In the long term, it is also extremely important to keep your adrenal glands healthy. Around the menopause, when the ovaries are beginning to produce less oestrogen, your body will need the oestrogen produced by the adrenal glands. This oestrogen helps to protect your bones and reduces the risk of osteoporosis.

Keeping your adrenals healthy

The first thing and most important step in boosting the health of your adrenals is to get your blood sugar in balance (see page 48). This will automatically prevent the release of some unnecessary adrenaline. It's also worth learning some form of relaxation, stress management technique or meditation, in order to help keep the effects of stress from damaging your body (see below). Take a careful look at your life, to see if there are any lifestyle factors involved. For example, if your job is simply too stressful, consider changing it. In the long run, your health will suffer if you are unable to adapt to and control the stress in your life. You may also find that psychotherapy or counselling is useful (see page 123). Or consider one of the many natural therapies now on offer, many of which are designed to encourage the body to cope better with stress, while learning to relax.

Some people need to be able to taught how to cope with stress. Women suffering from PMS may benefit in particular, for studies show that women with PMS use 'negative' coping strategies.[8] These can include:

- Overeating
- Overspending on shopping
- Alcohol dependency
- Tobacco or drug dependencies
- Watching too much television.

How to make changes

One of the most important aspects of stress reduction is making lifestyle changes. In a nutshell, stress is effectively anything that takes you up and over the 'healthy' threshold of stimulation and high energy. When things become too much – and this threshold will be different for every individual woman – symptoms such as irritability, sleep problems and digestive disorders will kick into action.

Every woman needs to learn to adapt her lifestyle in order to cope with or, better still, become resistant to stress. This involves ensuring that work pressures are reasonable, that you have time for yourself, that you eat well, get enough sleep, and, of course, exercise. It also means taking time for relaxation and leisure. Some women find it useful to book appointments with themselves to ensure that they make and take enough time to do things that they enjoy, including exercise, time with friends, or just a moment to be alone.

Exercise is vital. Studies show that it can reduce the impact of stress, raise self-esteem, relieve anxiety and depression, and improve mood, all of which are crucial for women who are suffering the symptoms of PMS.[9] Just three twenty-minute exercise sessions every week can make a big difference to overall health and wellbeing. And it's worth choosing something you enjoy, which apparently boosts the effectiveness of exercise as stress relief (see pages 78–86).

Sleep is also an important part of a healthy lifestyle, and far too many of us get too little. Stress and sleep are inversely related: the less sleep you get, the more difficult you'll find it to adapt to challenging situations. See pages 86–8 for more details.

As we saw in the last chapter, diet is extremely important. It affects every element of your life, and a healthy diet will give your body the tools it needs to perform at optimum level. Given the link between mind and body, it's clear that we will all feel better if we are physically well. Diet is the foundation of good health, and it can't be overestimated in relation to stress (see page 82).

There's more. Leisure time may be hard to find in your life, but it's essential to ensure relaxation and, most importantly, enjoyment. Having fun makes you feel better about yourself – more fulfilled, more satisfied, more interested and more engaged in the world outside that of your own personal experiences and concerns. There's an immense range of recreations. Some are quite demanding and even exhausting, such as playing tennis or squash, or cooking for friends, but they are all a source of pleasure and satisfaction and a chance to extend your skills. It's important merely that they're distinct from what you do at work, and don't involve any of your stress factors. If your stress arises mainly at the office, cooking at the weekend could be recreational – but if you spend hours in the kitchen already, that would be unlikely to be much fun.

Studies show that hobbies or leisure that involve other people provide social support that can help reduce stress even if the stressful situation remains unchanged. One study proved that people with fewer community ties were significantly more likely to die at a given age than those who had strong ties.[10]

Another aspect of coping with stress is learning to manage your time more effectively. Even if that means sitting down to plan out a weekly schedule, allowing yourself time with family and friends, and to relax doing something that you enjoy doing, it's worth the effort involved. If you take control of your time, you'll avoid falling into yet another stress trap – running late, missing appointments, eating on the run and never quite making time for yourself.

The only way to adapt to stress is to make changes that put you back in the driver's seat. You can regain this control – by downshifting, perhaps, changing jobs, making a decision to work at home, getting some extra help with the house or the children, refinancing, and putting the emphasis on your own health and wellbeing, rather than pouring energy into keeping up with the rat race. All this might seem a daunting prospect, but it's worth pursuing changes towards wellbeing. If you can keep your stress load down, and adapt to the stress you do face, you'll notice a marked difference in the way PMS symptoms affect you and your quality of life.

RELAXATION

As stress and the effects of adrenaline are known to play a major part in PMS, could learning to relax help with premenstrual symptoms? It has been found that relaxation therapy is helpful for PMS.[11] Another study showed that the use of progressive muscle relaxation followed by guided imagery has also proved effective in the treatment of this condition.[12] The latter technique also helped to lengthen short monthly cycles, which is relevant for many PMS sufferers. If you have short cycles, you will experience premenstrual symptoms much more frequently than necessary. With a 21-day cycle, for example, you could be suffering from PMS every two or three weeks, instead of every four or so, as is the case with the average 28-day cycle.

My recommendation is that anyone under stress should consider a form of relaxation, alongside the dietary recommendations and supplements suggested. Relaxation will mean something different for each woman. You may find it helpful to learn a structured relaxation technique. Here is the progressive muscle relaxation method mentioned in the research above.

1 Tense each part of your body as you breathe in. Then hold your breath for five seconds while you keep the muscles tense.

Relax and breathe out again slowly over a count of about ten seconds.

2 Curl your toes up and press down with your feet. Relax.
3 Press your heels down, pulling your toes up. Relax.
4 Tense your calf muscles. Relax.
5 Straighten your legs and tense your thigh muscles. Relax.
6 Tighten your buttocks. Relax.
7 Tighten your stomach muscles. Relax.
8 Bend your elbows up and flex your biceps. Relax.
9 Hunch your shoulders and tense your neck muscles. Relax.
10 Clench your teeth, frown and screw up your eyes as tight as you can. Relax.
11 Tense all your muscles at the same time. After ten seconds, relax.
12 Now close your eyes. Concentrate your mind on an imaginary diamond glinting on a black velvet background for thirty seconds as you continue to breathe slowly and deeply.
13 Now focus on another peaceful object of your choice for thirty seconds.
14 Now open your eyes.

Some women find that using a guided-imagery tape can help them focus their mind. Concentrating on the image of the diamond, as above, is one way of doing this.

A simple visualisation technique can also be useful. Simply imagine yourself on a beautiful beach or in a fragrant, colourful garden. Fully appreciate these imagined surroundings – feel the warm sun on your skin and the soft sand under your feet, and see the blue sky and the clear water. Smell different flowers, feel the fresh green grass, and hear the gurgle of a stream nearby. Choose your own paradise to enter for a few short minutes. Once you are inhabiting this place of peace and relaxation, you can choose to enter it at any time, anywhere. Taking the time to change your state of mind can feel totally refreshing.

Not only have relaxation techniques helped with PMS; they have also been found to be helpful for period pains.[13] After all, the womb is a muscle and any relaxation technique can benefit your whole body.

Stress and supplements

Certain nutrients, such as zinc, the B vitamins – especially B5 (pantothenic acid) and B6 (pyridoxine) – vitamin C and the essential fatty acids or EFAs, can be extremely helpful when stress is a problem, and they will help to optimise the functioning of the adrenal glands. See pages 173–4 for details of dosages and the treatment plan most appropriate for you.

If you are under a lot of stress, make sure you add in not just B vitamins and EFAs, but also vitamin C, which is not normally suggested for PMS. When you're stressed you excrete more vitamin C through urinating than at any other time. Smoking and pollution also deplete levels of this important antioxidant in your bloodstream. Vitamin C is vital for keeping your immune system strong, and when we fail to get enough of it we can be susceptible to any infections going around.

Natural remedies for stress

If stress is affecting your sleep (see pages 86–8), herbs can be very helpful. Valerian, a herbal sedative, is wonderful for helping with insomnia. Passion-flower or passiflora is another good herb for helping you sleep and can be used together with valerian for maximum effect. A cup of hot chamomile tea before bed can also help.

Herbs can support the adrenal glands, induce a sense of relaxation, and protect organs and systems under pressure. No adrenal gland treatment would be complete without Siberian ginseng (*Eleutherococcus senticosus*), which stands head and shoulders above the rest. This herb is classed as an adaptogen, which means that it works according to your body's needs, providing energy when required, and helping to combat stress and fatigue when you are under pressure. It helps to support adrenal gland function and acts as a tonic to these glands. Siberian ginseng is extremely useful when you have been under mental or physical stress, and should be taken for about three months for best effect.

Taking herbs that support your liver (see page 77) is a good idea, given the extra pressure placed on this organ by stress.

Aromatherapy oils such as bergamot, lavender and chamomile can be added to a relaxing warm bath just before you go to bed, and some women have said that essential oil of lavender sprinkled onto the pillow is restful. Massage can be either invigorating or relaxing, depending upon what you need. You can add any of the essential oils I've mentioned to a light 'carrier' oil such as grapeseed, and use it as often as possible in massage. Massage with aromatherapy oils has been shown to be helpful in the treatment of PMS.[14]

Oils that strengthen the action of the adrenals can be used in the short term, but you have to be careful about overuse. Good choices are geranium and rosemary. Rosemary is also a gentle stimulant, which can help to increase energy levels when you are experiencing stress. Sedative and anti-depressant oils that are noted for initiating the relaxation response include bergamot, clary sage, jasmine, marjoram and rose.

The therapeutic benefits of massage are well documented. Preliminary results of a study at the James Cancer Hospital and Research Institute in Columbus, Ohio, suggested that cancer patients had less pain and anxiety after receiving therapeutic massage. Women who had experienced the recent death of a child were less depressed after receiving therapeutic massage, according to preliminary results of a study at the University of South Carolina. Further studies have shown that massage improves wellbeing, and the functioning of the immune and nervous systems, and lowers stress hormone levels. They have also found that it can control cortisol levels, which are so affected by stress.[15]

There are many other natural therapies that have been successful in reducing stress. The World Health Organization recognises acupuncture as an appropriate treatment for stress and stress-related disorders, while reflexology, yoga and T'ai chi are widely used to help. The bottom line is to find a therapy that works for you, and stick with it. You may find the process of experimenting with the various treatments available relaxing in itself.

Sleep

Sleep is not only important for overall health, but essential for ensuring that your body is working at optimum levels, and that you are physically and emotionally able to cope with the demands of day-to-day life. Unfortunately, sleep problems are often associated with PMS, producing a bit of a double-whammy situation in which women who are less equipped to cope with lack of sleep find that they are having to bear bouts of sleeplessness.

Sleep gives your body time to recharge its batteries, repair tissues and grow cells. Most of us know what it's like to be sleep-deprived, with its associated feelings of irritability, poor concentration and lethargy. Most of these symptoms are controllable and acceptable on the odd occasion, but for many women, sleep disturbances occur every month as part of their premenstrual symptoms.

Yet however vital sleep is, we continue to chip away at the time we give to it. As a society, we have pushed the waking day to the limits, and sleep has become a luxury. Since the early 1900s, an average night's sleep has been reduced from 9 hours to about 7.5. Before the invention of electric light, people slept when it was dark because they were restricted by what could be done without light. Today, we can watch television 24 hours a day, shop in the middle of the night and surf the Net around the clock. Not only is it possible to undertake a wide range of activities during the day and night, but also we live in a state of information overload, in which there is enormous pressure to undertake as many things as possible. We are identified and judged by our achievements and our 'busyness'. Not surprisingly, we need to stay up later and later in order to fit it all in.

What does sleeplessness do to us? For some time scientists have questioned what happens to our metabolic and endocrine (hormone) functions when we are deprived of sleep. One important study in relation to PMS looked at the effects of inadequate sleep on blood sugar. The researchers based their findings on people who managed only four hours of sleep per night over six days.[16] It was found that after only six days of restricted sleep, the body's ability to secrete and respond to insulin, which helps to regulate blood sugar, had dropped by 30 per cent. The researchers claimed that this difference in glucose effectiveness is nearly identical to that reported between groups of patients with non-insulin-dependent diabetes – known as Type II – and normal people. It is well known that a decrease in acute insulin response to glucose is an early marker of diabetes (see page 163).[17]

Ultimately, then, a lack of sleep will make PMS worse, because it increases the blood sugar problems that are known to exacerbate the condition (see page 49). And in the long term, not getting enough sleep could actually make you more susceptible to Type II diabetes (see pages 163–4).

Scientists also looked at saliva samples of cortisol, which is one of the hormones released by the adrenal glands. Cortisol is important for the normal metabolism of carbohydrates, and for a healthy response to stress. Researchers found that when people are sleep-deprived, the rate at which cortisol is decreased in the body between the hours of 4 and 9 pm is some six times slower. What's more, the ageing process appears to be increased over this period.[18] So not only can lack of sleep increase your risk of late-onset diabetes, and worsen your PMS symptoms – it will also make you age more quickly.

The list goes on. Inadequate sleep also lowers the immune response. A recent study showed that missing even a few hours a night on a regular basis can decrease the number of the immune system's 'natural killer cells', which are responsible for fighting off invaders such as bacteria and viruses. This will come as no surprise to those of us who succumb to colds and other illnesses when we are run down – normally after periods of inadequate sleep.

Even occasional sleeping problems can make daily life feel more stressful or cause you to be less productive. In fact, inadequate sleep is associated with poor memory, an inability to make reasoned decisions and to concentrate, as well as irritability and, of course, fatigue. You may recognise many of these symptoms alongside other health complaints. The answer is to get to bed early, and ensure that you are sleeping well by following the tips below for getting a good night's sleep.

There are two main types of sleep problems:

- Finding it difficult getting off to sleep when you go to bed
- Falling off to sleep easily, but waking in the middle of the night and finding it difficult to get back to sleep again

It's more common for women with PMS to experience the latter problem.

Our physical and mental states are so intertwined that they constantly feed off one another. If something is worrying you mentally, your body can become tense and find it difficult to let go and relax. This makes sleep more difficult, which, of course, makes you feel more stressed. You worry that you are not sleeping, and are concerned about how you will cope the following day. And if you are experiencing physical symptoms, such as aches and pains, this can make you worried and agitated, causing more tension and feelings of stress. Not surprisingly, your sleep patterns could well end up disrupted.

Tips for a good night's sleep

1. Avoid any foods or drinks containing caffeine, such as tea, coffee, cola drinks and chocolate, during the day. The caffeine will act as a stimulant and make it harder for you to fall asleep. Everybody has a different sensitivity to caffeine, but for some women just one cup of coffee a day, even in the morning, is enough to prevent them from getting to sleep at night. Even decaffeinated coffee can be a problem because it contains other stimulants that can keep you awake.

2. Make sure that you are eating little and often during the day to keep your blood sugar steady. This will make sure that your adrenaline levels are steady and will help to prevent the adrenal glands from overworking. This in turn makes sure that the hormone cortisol, which is produced from the adrenals, starts to wind down when you go to bed, as it is supposed to do (see page 79).

3. If you regularly wake in the middle of the night – especially if you wake abruptly and with palpitations – have a small snack of complex carbohydrates, such as an oatcake or half a slice of wheat or rye bread about an hour before bed. This will stop your blood sugar from dropping overnight, and prevent adrenaline from being released into the bloodstream to try and correct this imbalance. This is called nocturnal hypoglycaemia.

4. Avoid alcohol. Not only does it affect blood sugar levels, which causes adrenaline to be released, but it also blocks the transport of tryptophan into the brain. Tryptophan is important because it is converted into serotonin, the calming and relaxing neurotransmitter (see page 42).

5. Have a cup of chamomile tea before bed, which will encourage relaxation.

6. When you exercise, try to do so early in the day. Exercise can be enormously stimulating, and some women may find it difficult to sleep following a late session. Furthermore, vigorous activity delays melatonin secretion (see page 121). If you exercise in the morning, you will reinforce healthy sleeping habits that lead to regular melatonin production.

7. Consider using some aromatherapy oils, such as bergamot, lavender, Roman chamomile and marjoram, in a warm bath just before bed. Avoid a hot bath, which can be stimulating, but ensure that it's warm enough to encourage relaxation. A few drops of aromatherapy oils on your pillow at bedtime, or used in a vaporiser, can have the same effect. A pre-bed, gentle massage with the same oils will help to encourage sleep.

8. Keep to a sleep routine, if possible setting your alarm for the same time each day. Many women fall into a poor and ultimately unsociable pattern, where they wake too early and struggle to stay awake in the evenings. Sometimes we need to reprogramme our body clocks to ensure not only that we are getting enough restful sleep, but that we are

getting it when we want to get it – in other words, at night! Once into a good routine, your body will respond by waking at the appropriate hour, and shutting down when you are tired in the evenings.

9. At least an hour before bed, write yourself a 'to do' list, so that you don't lie in bed mulling over what needs to be done as you go to sleep.

10. Making love can help you go to sleep by relaxing you, and releasing tension.

11. Herbs can be extremely helpful for sleep-related problems. Hops, passionflower and skullcap all work as gentle sedatives and can help you to overcome insomnia. Try not to rely on only one herb, but rotate among several, to ensure that you don't become overly dependent. And as we've seen, chamomile is another useful sedative, and it helps to calm and tone the nervous system, promoting restful sleep.

12. Magnesium, which is known as 'nature's tranquilliser', is good for helping with sleep problems. If you suffer from 'restless legs' or cramps, take both magnesium (250mg per day) and vitamin E (300iu per day).

13. Use visualisation techniques. Imagine yourself on a beautiful beach with the warm sun on your skin, soft sand under your feet, blue sky, clear water and the fragrant scent of wonderful coloured flowers. You could also have some soothing music playing while you let yourself go and imagine yourself in this tropical paradise. This technique is very useful if you have an active mind that simply won't switch off, even when you are physically tired. By focusing the mind on something which is relaxing, you will find it is much easier for the mind to 'let go'.

14. Learn to practise relaxation. Try lying on your back and, starting from your toes, tense each part of your body in turn and then relax. So curl and tense the toes, hold for a few seconds and then relax and repeat all the way up the body. Don't leave the head out: screw up your face and then release the muscles. This way you can actually feel the difference between tension and relaxation and you know what you are aiming for each time you relax. You could also use some relaxing music to go with this.

SLEEPING PILLS
It is better to avoid sleeping pills. They alter the natural cycles of deep and light sleep during the night. We have different stages of sleep (deep and light) and in the first two-thirds of the night, both stages occur. In the last third of the night, we experience only light sleep. REM (rapid eye movement) or 'dream' sleep occurs approximately every ninety minutes. All of these stages of sleep are equally important, and sleeping pills disrupt this cycle. If you are already taking sleeping pills you must see your doctor before stopping them.

Tryptophan

Tryptophan is an important amino acid for sleep problems because the body makes serotonin (the 'feelgood' brain chemical) from it. Tryptophan occurs naturally in foods such as dairy products, fish, bananas, dried dates, soya, almonds and peanuts. It is no longer available as a supplement (see page 106), but a new product, called 5-HTP, has taken its place.

5-HTP has been used in clinical trials to lessen the time it takes to get off to sleep and to stop the number of awakenings during the night.[19]

Warning: If you are taking mono-amine oxidase (MAOI) inhibitor drugs for depression, or any other drugs for depression, you should not take tryptophan.

Napping

It has been said that both Winston Churchill and Margaret Thatcher survived during office on small amounts of sleep at night because they took naps during the day. Some women find that this works very well, and that a short, ten- to fifteen-minute cat nap (or 'power' nap, as they are sometimes called) can relieve stress and renew energy.

Some women, however, claim that they feel worse after napping, or find that they simply can't sleep for short periods of time, and end up losing an hour or so a day in an attempt to get a short, refreshing rest.

The trick in napping is to fall asleep sitting up. If you go to bed or lie down the tendency is to go into a deeper sleep, which makes you feel groggy if you don't get enough – or sends you off to sleep for too long. According to some research, twenty-five minutes is the optimum time for a short nap.

Exercise

The benefits of regular exercise cannot be exaggerated, particularly when you suffer from PMS.

You may already know some of the benefits of exercise, such as the positive effect on your heart and circulation, and its ability to lower LDL ('bad' cholesterol) and increase HDL ('good' cholesterol) as well as helping to reduce high blood pressure. Exercise also helps to keep your bowels working efficiently, eliminating waste products that your body doesn't need. And it improves the functioning of the immune system and the lymph system, and helps to stimulate thyroid gland secretion to improve thyroid function. This has a direct effect on your metabolism and also helps to balance hormones produced by the thyroid gland while encouraging the body to use the hormones effectively.

But how does exercise affect PMS? Women who engage in moderate aerobic exercise at least three times a week have significantly fewer premenstrual symptoms than sedentary women.[20] Regular exercise also helps to improve your body's ability to keep your blood sugar in balance, which as we've seen is especially important in eliminating premenstrual symptoms.

Exercise releases brain chemicals called endorphins, which help us to feel happier, more alert and calmer.[21] These endorphins can have a dramatic and positive effect on the depression, stress and anxiety associated with PMS.

For all these reasons – relieving stress, boosting energy and creating a sense of wellbeing – exercise is now thought to be an essential part of any treatment for PMS.[22] But the type of exercise you choose can make a difference to how beneficial it will be in reducing premenstrual symptoms. When comparing aerobic exercise to strength training, it has been found that while both types of exercise help generally with premenstrual symptoms, aerobic exercise has the better effect on the most symptoms, particularly depression.[23]

And there's more. Exercise also send blood surging through the tissues, supplying them with energy-generating oxygen. It helps to eliminate waste, which could encourage water retention, headaches and irritability. And working up a sweat increases the circulation and helps to optimise the functioning of the lymphatic system.

One study looked at the effectiveness of exercise and of drugs in alleviating depression. The patients were split into three groups – exercise only, exercise and drugs, and drugs only. After a year, symptoms had returned in only 8 per cent of the patients who were exercising, compared to 38 per cent of the group who were taking drugs. And 31 per cent of the exercise-plus-drugs group relapsed. Just half an hour of brisk walking three times a week was enough to keep the symptoms at bay. The researchers were surprised that the exercise- and drugs-programme did not fare better than exercise on its own, as they assumed the effect would be additive. They believed that simply taking a pill is very passive, and that by exercising, the patients may have felt that they were taking an active role in getting better.[24]

As well as increasing endorphin levels, which helps with mood, exercise also seems to act as a stress-reliever and it is believed to lower excessively high cortisol levels (see pages 79–80).

Exercise is also crucial for the health of your bones, especially as you get older. It helps to maintain a good level of bone density, which could prevent osteoporosis after the menopause.

If that's not enough to convince you, consider this: it's now known that exercise can also have a direct effect on controlling your hormones, especially oestrogen. One fascinating study showed that women who exercised for around four hours a week had a 58 per cent lower risk of breast cancer, and those who routinely exercised for between one and three hours a week had a 30 per cent lower risk.[25] The thinking is that regular exercise modifies a woman's hormonal activity in a beneficial way. We know that extremes of exercise alter the menstrual cycle dramatically – many women athletes, for instance, don't have periods at all. So it is believed that moderate routine exercise suppresses the production, or overproduction, of hormones, reducing a woman's exposure during her lifetime. Some breast cancers are oestrogen-sensitive, so it makes sense that if the hormone levels are more balanced, the risk of developing breast cancer will be reduced.

In terms of PMS, this is a very interesting development. If exercise can help to keep hormones in balance, problems with inadequate production or use of progesterone may be minimised, as oestrogen will not be able to become overdominant.

Although exercise is good for us, beware taking it to extremes. As I've mentioned, your periods can stop if you exercise too often or too strenuously. In much the same way as crash dieting, overexercising can reduce your body fat to a level where menstruation ceases, as many female gymnasts and athletes know to their cost.

Over the years our lifestyles have changed, and we have become more sedentary. We have washing machines, most of us use the car to go shopping, and many of our jobs involve sitting behind a computer. So it's important as never before that we make time for exercise, to fit it into an already busy schedule. Don't be tempted to put it on the bottom of your to-do list. It's a priority for your health.

We should all try to make exercise a conscious part of our daily lives. It doesn't have to mean spending a lot of money on joining an expensive gym. You can use your daily routine to help you get the exercise you need. Instead of taking the lift, walk up the stairs. When you are on an escalator, walk instead of standing still. Run, rather than walk, up the stairs at home and deliberately park the car further away from the shops. None of us would want to go back to the days when the household jobs were an endless, demoralising grind of exhausting physical effort, but we all have to find some way of making up for the lack of everyday exercise in our lives.

As regular exercise is more beneficial than occasional bursts, it is best to find something you enjoy which will motivate you to do it regularly. Brisk walking is very beneficial and can be fitted in most times.

Choose an exercise that fits in with your family, lifestyle and finances. If you find something that you enjoy, such as dancing, tennis, yoga or swimming, you are more likely to continue doing it.

You may prefer to vary how you exercise so that you don't get bored. Remember that weight-bearing exercise, like walking, is the best for your bones. Try to do some every day.

> **GET SUPPORT**
>
> Make sure that you wear a good sports or support bra for exercising, especially during the premenstrual period. Your breasts can become fuller and heavier during this period, and you will need to support the breast tissue when you become more active.

CHAPTER 7

Food Supplements

You may wonder whether it's really necessary to take supplements, particularly if you have a good diet. Surely a healthy, varied diet will supply everything you need?

Unfortunately, the answer is no. The well-balanced diet is a myth, and the vast majority of us will not get all the nutrients we need from our food. This was confirmed in a National Food Survey conducted in 1995, which found that the average person in Britain is grossly deficient in six out of the eight vitamins and minerals surveyed. Fewer than one in ten people receive the Recommended Daily Allowance of zinc, which is the most important mineral for female hormone problems.

No matter how good your diet, or your intentions, it is virtually impossible to get all the nutrients from food alone. For instance, our daily intake of selenium (34mcg) is now only half of what it was just twenty-five years ago. And our current daily intake is just half the minimum 75mcg a day recommended for men and the 60mcg recommended for women.

For your food to contain the nutrients it needs, the soil on which it is grown needs to be rich in nutrients. For instance, carrots will extract the minerals from the soil and you absorb the nutrients when you eat them. But our soil has been overfarmed, and pesticides and other chemicals have been used to the point where the soil itself simply does not contain the quantity of nutrients we require.

Furthermore, our modern diet tends to be based on a great deal of processed, convenience and refined foods that have been stripped of essential nutrients through the manufacturing process. For example, 80 per cent of zinc is removed from wheat during the milling process to ensure that a loaf of bread, for instance, has a longer shelf life.[1] And there are other problems with our modern diet. Many chemicals used in producing it (and that includes pesticides and other treatments used in farming of even healthy foods) act as 'anti-nutrients', meaning that our bodies need more of the basic nutrients in order to process them into a usable form. So rather than adding vitamins, minerals and other essential elements to our bodies, the modern diet actually uses up vital nutrients that may already be there.

You can also be deficient in certain nutrients if you have been dieting for a number of years, either restricting your food intake or trying different diet drinks or pills.

But how can supplements help with PMS? The fact is that certain supplements can help to speed up the process of eliminating premenstrual symptoms because they can help you to detoxify, balance your hormones or blood sugar, or just ensure that your body is working at its optimum level.

It is important, however, to remember that supplements are just what their name suggests – supplemental, or 'extra'. They are not a substitute for healthy food and a well-balanced diet. You cannot eat junk food and take nutritional supplements and hope to stay healthy.

A word on the best nutrients for PMS

A number of nutrients have been studied in relation to PMS, including calcium, magnesium, vitamin E, vitamin B6 and also evening primrose oil. But remember, too, that women with PMS have shown a high placebo response (see page 43) and that this happens whether scientists are testing a drug or a nutrient.

The placebo effect is often seen as an indication of something irrational, but would it be possible to enhance the placebo effect by seeing how it works? Hippocrates, the Greek 'father of medicine', talked about the 'self-healing' process. This process works on the premise that given the right tools, the body can heal and balance itself. Health has been defined as a concept that 'involves recognition of the body as having self-regulatory, self-defending, self-repairing and cell replicatory capabilities'.[2]

Is it possible that the placebo – or perhaps we should call it the old 'bedside manner' – is a catalyst of this self-healing, self-regulatory process? The placebo response is short-lived. Although one study showed that in women with PMS it can be as high as 94 per cent, it did only last for a month or so. Yet perhaps this concept could be helpful as a starting point for treatment. Women with PMS have often been to a number of different specialists, often with no relief, because with 150 possible symptoms, misdiagnosis is all too common.

Women often say to me that they go to their doctor with what they call their 'shopping list' of symptoms, but because the doctors are under such time pressures, women very rarely have enough time to explain what is happening. When these same women are examined for the purposes of a clinical trial, they will have someone taking the time to explain what the trial involves and how it all works. What's more, their problems will be acknowledged and noted, and their symptoms will then be assessed over a couple of months to confirm a PMS diagnosis. The placebo response can actually kick into action at the beginning of the trial, largely because these women are given due care and attention, which may well be one of the mechanisms that begins the self-healing process. If the correct treatment is not given, this process wanes.

But although both drug and supplement studies can show a placebo effect, there are enormous differences between the drug approach and the nutritional approach. Drugs will only work when you are taking them, and will do absolutely nothing to correct the underlying problem. When you stop taking them, your PMS symptoms will return. The drugs do not change your underlying general health.

The aim of the natural approach is to correct any vitamin and mineral deficiencies, as well as making sure that you are eating well. It also involves using herbs and other supplements to ensure that your body is working effectively. The idea is that you change and optimise your overall health, so that the way your body responds to outside stimuli (such as stress) and the way it responds to its own ups and downs (such as your monthly cycle) is fundamentally different. It is possible to cure PMS in the long term, without having to rely on a treatment that needs to be taken every month.

I will show you which of the nutrients are most effective in the treatment of PMS, and help you to work out a dose that will work for you. Most studies are based around giving a standard dose of a nutrient – let's say, vitamin B6. The drawback of this approach is that all women are unique, and their requirements for any nutrient will be dramatically different. Unless the dosage is correct, there can be little or no effect.

At the end of this chapter, I suggest a programme of supplements for you to follow over a period of three to six months, which not only will enhance the dietary benefits described in Chapter 5, but will take into consideration a number of other issues that will make the programme much more effective.

Katherine

Katherine was thirty-four when she came to see me. She already had two daughters aged five and six, but she wanted to have another child. She didn't, however, think that she would ever be well enough to contemplate becoming pregnant again.

She had breastfed both of her daughters, during which time she suffered night sweats. After the birth of her second daughter, she was put on the Pill. Two years later, she was put on a different Pill, which caused her to develop ovarian cysts which grew and then burst. She then started to suffer from headaches and became very anxious. Her gynaecologist told her that it was a lack of oestrogen. The Pill was stopped and she was given oestrogen patches to use for two weeks in the month. She started to get dizzy spells, aches and pains, and pins and needles in her feet. She felt extremely tired and was spotting on days 14 and 15 of her cycle.

All of these symptoms (except the spotting) fluctuated with her cycle, becoming worse in the second half. At this time, the anxiety was so severe that her GP put her on Prozac. Her doctor claimed that she was clinically depressed, while her gynaecologist believed her problem to be a lack of oestrogen. By this time Katherine was at her wits' end – and she had two young children to look after. When she came to see me she had stopped the Prozac and was back on the Pill. That month, she had been bleeding continuously since day 10 of her cycle.

We discussed the fact that the ultimate aim was to get her back to optimum health. To do this we would ensure that she was eating well and that any vitamin and mineral deficiencies were corrected. She mentioned that when she got anxious she would start to shake and then have a teaspoon of sugar. She had been tested for diabetes, but the test proved to be negative. I explained how blood sugar levels could cause what seemed like psychological symptoms, such as mood swings, anxiety and depression.

A hair mineral analysis showed that she was severely deficient in zinc and had high copper levels, which usually results from taking the Pill or any reproductive hormones. I put her on a programme to redress the zinc/copper imbalance, balance her blood sugar fluctuations and support her adrenal glands. Katherine also decided to stop taking the Pill.

Katherine came back the following month to say that she had not any spotting for the first time in three and a half years. She was also pleased to find that her bowel movements had become more regular, which had also not occurred for over ten years. Her energy had improved dramatically and she was starting to feel more like her 'old self'. That was two years ago. Katherine now has a daughter of eight months, whom she is still breastfeeding – with no night sweats!

Vitamin B6 (pyridoxine)

There have been many studies showing the effectiveness of vitamin B6 on PMS. It was first used for hormone imbalances in the 1970s when it was used in the treatment of depression caused by the Pill.[3] The latest review, published in 1999 in the *British Medical Journal*, showed that daily doses of 100mg, or even 50mg, of vitamin B6, were twice as effective as the placebo treatment.[4] Some concerns had previously been raised about high doses of B6 causing tingling in the hands and feet, but this review found no evidence of any side-effects for doses of 100mg or less per day.

The majority of research has shown that vitamin B6 makes a substantial difference across the whole range of PMS symptoms, but some studies have shown no benefit. It has been suggested that this could be due to the fact that vitamin B6 was given on its own.

We know that all the vitamins and minerals are 'synergistic', which means that they work together. No matter what other supplements you choose to take you should always make a good multivitamin and mineral supplement the foundation of your programme (see page 108). This ensures that all of the vitamins, minerals and trace elements in the entire spectrum are present, so that any interdependent actions can take place.

In order for your body to convert B6 (as pyridoxine), into its active form, pyridoxal-5-phosphate, which your body can use, it needs other nutrients such as magnesium. So if you take B6 on its own, but have other (even small) nutritional deficiencies, your body may not be able to use the B6 properly. It is also possible to buy vitamin B6 in the form of pyridoxal-5-phosphate instead of pyridoxine in the event that your body has any problems making the conversion to the active form.

Vitamin B6 plays a vital part in synthesising certain brain chemicals called neurotransmitters, which control your mood and behaviour. It is required as a co-enzyme in the production of dopamine, tryptophan and serotonin. When treating the depressive symptoms of PMS, it is important that nutrients known to affect serotonin production, such as B6, are taken in adequate quantities. Prozac, for example, is used in the treatment of depression and also now for PMS (see page 42) and it is called a selective serotonin re-uptake inhibitor (SSRI) because it optimises the use of serotonin.

Vitamin B3 (niacin)

This is an important vitamin for eliminating premenstrual symptoms because it is needed for enzyme formation and involved in both glucose and carbohydrate metabolism. Vitamin B3 is also needed for the proper regulation of blood sugar.

Vitamin B5 (pantothenic acid)

Like vitamin B3, vitamin B5 is involved in energy production, but it also optimises the functioning of the adrenal glands. It is an important vitamin in PMS because of its anti-stress effects. One of the signs of a severe deficiency is the 'burning foot syndrome', in which it feels as if your feet are on fire.

More on the Bs

The B vitamins are called the 'stress' vitamins because of their ability to help us cope with the pressures of everyday life. Many of them, such as B2, B3 and B6, are needed for normal thyroid hormone production. Poor thyroid function has been implicated in PMS (see pages 159–62), so it is very important to ensure that your thyroid gland is functioning optimally. The B vitamins are also key because of their effect on the liver (see page 77), helping it to clear out 'old' hormones, a process crucial in proper detoxification.

The B vitamins are also important for the conversion of linoleic acid to gamma-linolenic acid or GLA, which is necessary to produce the beneficial prostaglandins (see page 61). As I discussed in Chapter 5, linoleic acid is an essential fatty acid found in foods such as corn oil, fresh nuts and seeds, and safflower oil. It's also known as an omega 6 oil. The B vitamins are required to convert this essential oil into a form that can be used by the body to produce 'good' types of prostaglandins. Without this conversion, our bodies would produce more of the 'bad' prostaglandins, which can increase PMS symptoms.

Vitamin E

This vitamin is helpful for breast symptoms associated with PMS, and also for mood swings and irritability.[5] It is interesting that women with PMS have not been found to be deficient in vitamin E[6] and yet it seems to help with the symptoms. At the moment, nobody is sure how it is working.

NATURAL OR SYNTHETIC VITAMIN E?

With most vitamins, the natural and synthetic forms are equal in effect because their molecular structures are identical. Of course, we should aim to take supplements that are closest to what we normally eat in our diet. Vitamin E, however, is completely different – the structures of its natural and synthetic forms are not the same. Scientists have studied the two forms to see how they influence the workings of our bodies. They have found that natural vitamin E is more biologically active than the synthetic version, which means that the body will utilise the natural form more easily. It is also retained in the body tissue for longer, which enables it to perform its protective effects in the long term.

When you buy vitamin E, choose the natural version, which is known as d-alpha-tocopherol. Avoid the synthetic version, dl-alpha-tocopherol.

Magnesium

This mineral is classed as 'nature's tranquilliser' and is very important in treating PMS, especially symptoms such as anxiety, tension and other negative emotional states. Women with PMS have been found to have lower levels of red blood cell magnesium than women who don't suffer symptoms.[7] Giving magnesium supplements has been found to be extremely useful in alleviating many PMS symptoms, and even more effective when taken with vitamin B6.[8] The two work together in many enzyme systems in the body, and it is said that B6 allows magnesium to enter cells and so helps to increase amounts of the mineral within them.

Magnesium does not just alleviate emotional symptoms, but also helps with fluid retention.[9] This includes swollen fingers and ankles, weight gain, breast tenderness and abdominal bloating.

Magnesium also aids in the production of insulin and helps to regulate blood sugar levels, which are, as we've now abundantly seen, crucial for eliminating premenstrual symptoms.

The mineral can help with migraines, too. During a migraine attack the blood vessels around the brain constrict, then dilate. This dilation is thought to cause migraine pain. A magnesium deficiency can cause blood vessels to go into spasm, so it could increase the risk of dilation. One study where magnesium was given to menstrual migraine sufferers found that it helped with not only the intensity but also the duration of the migraines.[10]

As I've noted elsewhere, magnesium deficiency isn't easy to test for. It only shows up if red blood cells are tested because both plasma and serum magnesium levels are a crude measure of magnesium and are usually normal.[11] So we can't put any real faith in studies stating that women with PMS do not have a magnesium deficiency, particularly when they are testing their blood in the wrong way.[12]

As you can see from all of the above, magnesium is something of a marvel, and it's vital to ensure your levels are optimal. Nor does the story end there. Magnesium also helps to increase aldosterone, a hormone released by the adrenal glands and which acts on the kidneys to regulate water balance, and decreases the neurotransmitter dopamine. So a magnesium deficiency could explain the water retention, depression and anxiety associated with PMS.

Calcium

For the last fifty years it has been known that irritability, anxiety, fatigue, depression, impaired memory and muscle cramps are associated with hypocalcaemia (low calcium levels), so one group of researchers decided to look at how giving calcium affected women with PMS. A total of 466 women took part in the trial and they were given either calcium or a placebo. The women were asked to rate the following symptoms: negative moods, water retention, food cravings and pain. By the third cycle, the women being given calcium experienced a 48 per cent reduction in all four symptoms, as compared to 30 per cent in the placebo group.[13]

Further research then looked at what happens to calcium levels over the menstrual cycle. In both women with PMS and those without, calcium levels vary through the month, with a significant drop around ovulation. But in the women with PMS, the mid-cycle parathyroid hormone (which increases blood calcium levels) was higher than in women without PMS. It was also found that women with PMS had lower vitamin D concentrations.[14]

What does this mean in practice? It indicates that women with PMS have disturbances in the way their bodies regulate calcium during their cycles.

Vitamin D is important because it stimulates the absorption of calcium. Without good levels of vitamin D, the body cannot absorb calcium from food or supplements, no matter how much you are getting. That is why having a good multivitamin and mineral (see page 108) is so important. It will give you a good foundation of all the nutrients, including vitamin D.

It seems calcium might be implicated in menstrual migraines, which have been relieved by giving a combination of the mineral and vitamin D.[15]

Zinc

Zinc is an important mineral because it is a component of more than 200 enzymes. It helps the conversion of linoleic acid to GLA (see page 61) and also plays a major part in the proper action of many of our hormones, including the sex hormones and insulin. Women with PMS have been found to have lower levels of zinc.[16]

Chromium

Chromium is needed for the metabolism of sugar, and without it insulin is less effective in controlling blood sugar levels. It helps insulin take glucose into the cells. In PMS, where many of the symptoms are similar to those of blood sugar imbalance, it is crucial that you have enough of this nutrient. Without enough chromium, glucose levels get higher because insulin's action is blocked. Insulin brings down the level of glucose.

It is now known that the average Western diet is deficient in chromium, and that two out of every three people suffers from hypoglycaemia, pre-hypoglycaemia or diabetes.[17]

Chromium is the most widely researched mineral used in the treatment of overweight, as it helps to control cravings and reduces hunger. Chromium also helps to control fat and cholesterol in the blood. One study showed that people who took chromium over a ten-week period lost an average of 1.9kg (4.2lb) of fat, while those on a placebo lost only 0.2kg (0.4lb).[18]

Chromium's effect on cravings is especially important if one of your main premenstrual symptoms involves shifts in appetite. Some women find that they can eat a packet of biscuits or a box of chocolates a day in the lead-up to their periods, while they would not think of eating like that at any other time of the month.

Ideally, chromium should be naturally present in the grains that you eat, such as wheat, corn, rye, oats, etc. However, as soon as these grains are refined, turned into white bread, pastries, biscuits and even pasta, for example, the chromium goes missing. So these refined carbohydrates are doubly problematic: they contribute to blood sugar imbalance because not only are they digested too fast, but also they lack the very mineral that would have helped balance blood sugar.

It is now thought that a chromium deficiency may play a major part in the increasing problem of hypoglycaemia, diabetes and obesity[19] and that because of our refined diet, many people now have lower levels of chromium than they should.[20]

> **Warning:** If you are diabetic, you need to speak to your doctor before supplementing with chromium.

Manganese

This mineral helps with the metabolism of fats, and also works to stabilise your blood sugar levels. It functions in many enzyme systems, including those enzymes involved in burning energy and in thyroid hormone function.

Essential fatty acids (EFAs)

We've already encountered these crucial fats (see pages 59–60). EFAs are necessary aids in the elimination of premenstrual symptoms, and should be included in your diet. But while you're waiting for the benefits of these to take effect, you should also take them in supplement form.

The omega 6 series of EFAs (see page 61), linoleic acid, is converted to gamma-linolenic acid (GLA), which is found in plants such as evening primrose, borage and starflower. But many women with PMS have been found to have a problem making this conversion to GLA because they lack an enzyme called delta-6-desaturase.[21] There are a number of factors that can prevent the conversion of linoleic acid into GLA, including stress, a high-sugar diet, and deficiencies of B6, magnesium and zinc. Because of this problem with conversion it is important to supplement these EFAs in the form where the conversion has already taken place – in other words, in the form of GLA. (The supplement label will actually say GLA rather than evening primrose oil or starflower oil, for example.)

A lot of research has centred around evening primrose oil (EPO) and its effects on PMS. Some have shown that it is effective in reducing the symptoms of PMS[22] whereas others have shown that it is no more effective than a placebo. The interesting point is that the best results with EPO occurred when women were also taking either B6 or a multivitamin,[23] which again confirms that supplements should not be taken in isolation.

Research has also shown that EPO may be most helpful to women whose main premenstrual symptom is breast tenderness or fibrocystic breast disease (see page 141).[24] It is usually needs to be taken for about three months to be effective, so don't give up.

Warning: Do not take evening primrose oil if you are epileptic.

Tryptophan

As we saw in Chapter 6, tryptophan is an amino acid with a vital effect on depression – the body uses it to make serotonin, the 'feelgood' brain chemical. Tryptophan occurs naturally in foods such as dairy products, fish, bananas, dried dates, soya, almonds and peanuts.

It is known that levels of serotonin are reduced in some women with PMS[25] and the new approach to PMS is to use antidepressants called SSRIs (selective serotonin re-uptake inhibitors, such as Prozac) to help control the symptoms. So it's now generally thought that we should keep serotonin levels at their optimum. The manufacture of serotonin depends on how much tryptophan is transported into the brain.

Tryptophan is only one of a number of amino acids, and the way you eat can determine how much tryptophan reaches your brain. Protein is made up of long chains of amino acids. When you eat protein, your body breaks it down into its different amino acids, which then travel into your bloodstream to reach your brain. There is a blood–brain barrier that controls what gets into your brain, so a competition starts to take place. There are fewer tryptophan molecules than there are of the other amino acids. Therefore, other amino acids get across the barrier, leaving the tryptophan behind.

If you eat carbohydrate with the protein, the situation is very different. Carbohydrates help the body release insulin, and insulin makes use of the other amino acids, leaving the tryptophan to dominate.

This is another reason why it is important that you do not follow a protein-only diet (see pages 56–7), and why combining protein and carbohydrates in one meal can be beneficial for PMS symptoms.

It is interesting that when we are feeling depressed we tend to want to eat bread, cakes, sweets and sugary foods, all of which are carbohydrates. In a sense, the body is trying to prescribe its own medication. It's right in doing so, and it's also right to follow your instincts, and the messages from your body. However, what is important here is the *type* of carbohydrate. As we've seen, healthy, whole carbohydrates provide a sustained release of energy, while refined foods cause a rise in insulin and blood sugar fluctuations.

I mentioned in the last chapter that tryptophan is no longer available as a supplement. L-tryptophan used to be available, but unfortunately, a Japanese biotech company produced a genetically engineered tryptophan that was implicated in thirty-seven deaths. A new product called 5-hydroxytryptophan (5-HTP), which comes from a small African bean called *Griffonia simplicifolia*, is now available instead. The bean had attracted the attention of scientists because in the body the 5-HTP converts naturally to the brain neurotransmitter serotonin (see also the effects of tryptophan on insomnia on page 91).

In fact, the 5-HTP has now been proved to be better than L-tryptophan and can also be taken with food, as it is not affected by other amino acids and can easily cross the blood-brain barrier.[26]

There has been a lot of research into the benefits of 5-HTP on depression, and it has been shown to be as effective as pharmaceutical antidepressants, but with fewer side-effects.[27] The researchers found '5-HTP and fluvoxamine [an antidepressant drug] to be distinctly effective in the treatment of depression and moreover to be equally so. Regarding tolerance and safety, however, 5-HTP proved superior to fluvoxamine as was apparent in a marked difference in the severity of untoward side-effects ... 'Our results strongly confirm the efficacy of 5-HTP as an antidepressant.'

Warning: If you are taking mono-amine oxidase (MAOI) inhibitor drugs for depression or any other drugs for depression, you should not take 5-HTP.

Antioxidants

Antioxidants are important substances that are contained naturally in the food we eat. They have a dramatic impact on overall health, mainly because they protect the body from the effects of substances known as 'free radicals'.

Oxygen, which is vital for our survival, can also be chemically reactive. It can become unstable, resulting in the 'oxidation' of other molecules, a process that in turn generates free radicals. Free radicals are a rather complicated concept, but in a nutshell, they are chemically unstable atoms that can cause all sorts of damage in your body. Pollution, smoking, fried or barbecued food and UV rays from the sun can also trigger these free radicals.

Free radicals have now been linked to health problems such as cancer, coronary heart disease and premature ageing. They speed up the ageing process by destroying healthy cells and they can also attack DNA in the nucleus of a cell, causing cell change, or mutation, and cancer. We have protection against free radicals in the form of antioxidants, which occur naturally in the food that we eat, especially in fruits and vegetables. Vitamins A, C and E, plus the minerals selenium and zinc, are all antioxidants and are contained in the following foods:

Sources of antioxidants

Vitamin A	Orange and yellow fruits and vegetables, such as carrots, pumpkins and oily fish
Vitamin C	Fruits (particularly citrus), green leafy vegetables such as broccoli, cauliflower, berries, potatoes and sweet potatoes
Vitamin E	Nuts, avocados, seeds, vegetable oils and oily fish
Selenium	Brazil nuts, tuna, cabbage
Zinc	Pumpkin and sunflower seeds, fish, almonds

It is known that both vitamin E and zinc have a direct impact on premenstrual symptoms (see pages 100–1 and 103), and all of the antioxidants help to keep you healthy. Your ultimate aim in treating PMS is to improve your overall health so that your body produces the correct amounts of hormones, and then uses those hormones exactly as nature intended over the cycle. Having good amounts of these antioxidants in your diet will help your body to do just that.

How to take supplements

Certain nutrients have been tested in isolation and found to be helpful for PMS. But what about all the others that have not been tested, such as selenium and manganese? In my opinion, individual vitamins and minerals do not need to be tested. As they work in harmony and most of them are dependent on each other to act efficiently, nutrients can't be tested in isolation because scientists will never get a true picture of what is really happening.

When you take any supplements, always ensure that a multivitamin and mineral forms the foundation of your regime. This will provide a good range of nutrients to prevent a fundamental imbalance that can be caused by taking supplements on their own. To this, add any extra supplements of the particular nutrients that are particularly beneficial for PMS.

When it comes to buying supplements, you get what you pay for. You will need good quality supplements for maximum absorption. I would recommend you buy capsules (preferably vegetable ones instead of gelatine) rather than tablets. Capsules tend to be filled only with the essential nutrients. Tablets can include a variety of fillers, binders and bulking agents.

Mineral supplements such as calcium should be taken in the form of citrates, ascorbates or polynicotinates, which are more easily absorbed by the body. Chlorides, sulphates, carbonates and oxides should be avoided as they are not so easily assimilated, and mineral supplements in this form may pass through the body without being absorbed. It is important to read the labels.

The other way that minerals are made more digestible is by chelation – pronounced *keylation* – where the mineral is 'hooked' onto an amino acid. This allows assimilation that is three to ten times greater than with non-chelated minerals. Choose chelated brands wherever possible.

Remember that cheaper versions are much less likely to be effective. Stick with well-established, reputable brands such as BioCare, Solgar, Lamberts and also The Natural Health Practice, who have an excellent product containing all the above nutrients as well as the herbs that follow in the next section.

For the correct dosages for all these important vitamins and minerals, see Chapter 13.

If you are already taking supplements and you want to know how well they are being absorbed, do the following test. Place your supplement in a glass of warm vinegar for thirty minutes, stirring every few minutes. The warm vinegar roughly represents the conditions found in your gut. If the supplement does not dissolve after half an hour, then, as the critics say, 'you are paying an awful lot for nutritious urine'. In other words, your nutrients are probably coming out the other end in much the same form that they entered! My recommendation would be to buy another brand.

And finally – take any vitamins and minerals with food. You want your body to think they are part of your diet, so that they are better absorbed along with your snacks or meals.

CHAPTER 8

Herbs

Herbs are the oldest form of medicine and have been used for healing in every culture in the world since the very beginning of recorded history at least, and probably much further back. Wise women have always played a central role in traditional cultures, and knowledge about herbs was passed on from one generation to the next. In fact, until the 19th century at least 90 per cent of all medicines were herbal.

Herbs are also the foundation of numerous pharmaceutical drugs. Aspirin is based on an extract from willow, originally used for pain relief by Native Americans. Up to 70 per cent of drugs in use today have their origins in plants, but Western pharmaceutical practice bears no relation to how native peoples the world over have used them. Modern drug companies only use the active ingredient of the plant or herb in a pure form as the basis for the drug. Ancient peoples used the whole plant, and the traditional cultures that have survived continue to do so. The advantage of using the whole plant is that the side-effects are absent or minimal. That is the big difference between modern and herbal medicine.

Take foxglove (*Digitalis purpurea*). Centuries ago it was used for heart problems. In modern times, scientists have isolated the main active ingredient of the foxglove, digoxin, and put it into tablet form. But by doing so, they have created a product with a real risk of side-effects. By the use of the whole plant, the active ingredient interacts with all the other constituents of the plant, which naturally contains 'buffer' ingredients that counteract any potential side-effects. Herbalists believe this is the proper way to use the healing powers of herbs and plants.

The easiest and most effective way to take herbs is in tincture form, using approximately 5ml (1 teaspoon) three times daily in a little water. Try to get tinctures made from organically grown herbs, which will not contain pesticides or any other toxic ingredients. In the liquid form, herbs are already dissolved, and so can be absorbed, and therefore work, more quickly.

Dried herbs, in tablets or capsules, have to be digested and, once again, they will work only to the extent that your body is able to process and absorb them. Herbs are not like drugs. If drugs are stopped, the symptoms can return and you are back where you started. Herbs may be aimed at easing symptoms, but they work at a more fundamental level and address the root of the problem as well as the symptoms. As your body becomes more balanced, the symptoms will begin to disappear.

Herbs that work best on premenstrual symptoms correct any hormone imbalances. Because no one is sure exactly which hormones are out of balance, it is better to take those that have a general balancing effect. I have also included some herbs for water retention, which may be helpful if you experience bloating or even breast tenderness. Other herbs suggested help support the liver, which detoxifies and excretes 'old' hormones.

In Chapter 13, you'll find details of the correct dosages, and the optimum duration of treatment, for each of these herbs.

Hormone-balancing herbs

I have listed these by the most commonly recognised name of each plant.

Vitex agnus-castus (Chasteberry tree)

Vitex agnus-castus, a violet-flowered fruit, is a member of the verbena family that grows around the Mediterranean and Central Asia. Hippocrates mentions it as beneficial for the female reproductive system. It was originally used by the ancient Greeks and Romans to decrease sex drive in men, especially monks – hence the name 'chasteberry' – but in fact may have the opposite effect on women's libido.

This is the most important herb in the treatment of PMS. It has been widely studied in relation to premenstrual symptoms and has been shown to be extremely helpful in re-establishing a normal balance of hormones. The latest research confirming the benefits of agnus-castus with PMS was reported in the *British Medical Journal* in 2001.[1] Over half the women taking the agnus-castus had a 50 per cent or greater improvement in symptoms, an effect that was experienced in just three cycles. The research concluded that 'agnus-castus is a well tolerated and effective treatment for the premenstrual syndrome, the effects being confirmed by physicians and patients alike. The effects are detected in most main symptoms of the syndrome.'

Agnus-castus helps to balance the sex hormones by working on the pituitary gland. It reduces follicle-stimulating hormone (FSH) and increases the production of luteinising hormone (LH), which then helps to balance the ratio of oestrogen to progesterone, particularly in the second half of the cycle. It is also helpful for water retention and may have a beneficial effect on the thyroid. And it seems to help where high levels of prolactin are a problem.[2]

Black cohosh (*Cicimicifuga racemosa*)

This herb is a good normaliser for the female reproductive system and can be useful for PMS. It was originally used by northern Native Americans, hence the other name by which it is known: squawroot. It has a generally calming effect on the nervous system and, as well as having a balancing effect on the hormones, it can be helpful when your main symptoms include anxiety, tension and depression. This would also be the herb to try if you get premenstrual headaches and cramps, as it has antispasmodic actions. It is well known as a powerful painkiller and is often useful as a preparation for giving birth. It is better to avoid this herb if you have heavy periods, and it should not be used in early pregnancy.

Skullcap (*Scutelleria lateriflora*)

Skullcap is a wonderful herb for the nervous system, and it is especially helpful if you experience anxiety, tension, depression, irritability, headaches and insomnia in the lead-up to your period. It also has antispasmodic qualities, which means that it can help with painful periods as well as aiding liver function.

Dong quai (*Angelica sinensis*)

Dong quai is a tall plant with branched leaves and white-green flowers. The root is used medicinally. The plant normally takes about three years before it is ready for harvest.

This Chinese herb has been in use since ancient times. It is a very popular for problems associated with the female reproductive system and is known as the 'female ginseng'. It can be helpful for PMS symptoms because it promotes normal hormone balance.[3] Dong quai also has muscle-relaxing qualities, so it is particularly suggested for women who experience premenstrual pain and cramps.[4]

In traditional Chinese medicine, dong quai is not used on its own, but combined with other herbs to give an overall beneficial effect. It is, however, known as the ultimate female 'tonic'.

Dong quai appears to have phytoestrogenic (see pages 66–8) effects,[5] which are extremely useful for problems such as PMS, where science has not yet come up with a cause. Phytoestrogens can be effective when the problem is caused by both too little *and* too much oestrogen. If oestrogen is low, they can exert a weak oestrogenic effect (about 400 times weaker than animal oestrogens), but if oestrogen is too high they can latch onto oestrogen receptors in the body and prevent extra oestrogen from going in.

The herb can also help to regulate blood sugar levels, which as we've seen is vital in PMS.

Herbs for water retention

As you change your eating patterns and approach optimum health, water retention will start to correct itself. You may, however, need some extra help at the beginning. Make sure that you reduce your intake of salt and salty foods. It's also important to drink more water. If you limit your intake of water your body will think there is a shortage and try to retain what little you take in. Water is a natural diuretic.

Dandelion (*Taraxacum officinale*)

Dandelion is the herb of choice for water retention because it is a natural diuretic, allowing fluid to be released without the body losing vital nutrients at the same time. It contains more vitamins and minerals than any other herb and is one of the best sources of potassium. Dandelion also helps to improve liver function, so it can be useful for general detoxification and elimination of hormones.

Many women who suffer from water retention turn to diuretics. When chemical diuretics are used, however, important minerals such as potassium may be lost. Dandelion is a perfect alternative: not only is it a powerful diuretic, but it contains good levels of potassium, which is crucial for the correct functioning of the heart.

The whole of the dandelion plant can be used therapeutically. The leaves have the greatest diuretic effect, while the root has a stronger action on the liver. This is one example of how using a whole plant rather than just parts can be important.

Dandelion also helps the pancreas work more effectively. It is the pancreas that secretes insulin, so dandelion can have a beneficial effect on balancing blood sugar levels.

Herbs for your liver

Your liver needs to be working efficiently in order to eliminate hormones and waste products. Furthermore, this vital organ can help to eliminate 'old' hormones safely and efficiently during each cycle. When you are trying to keep your hormones in balance, you do not want 'old' circulating hormones adding to the problem.

If you suffer from premenstrual or menstrual migraines or headaches, it is even more important that your liver is functioning efficiently. The liver filters the blood and removes toxins, pollutants, hormones and waste products. If these substances are not effectively removed from the blood, they can leave you feeling tired, depressed, lethargic and headachy.

Dandelion (*Taraxacum officinale*)

Once again dandelion steps to the fore – it's not just an excellent diuretic, but also has a therapeutic effect on the liver.

Milk thistle (*Silybum marianum*)

Milk thistle is a native of Western and Central Europe, but grows wild all over the world. It is a member of the daisy family and grows up to ten feet tall with purple flowers. The seeds of the plant are used therapeutically.

Milk thistle is an excellent herb for the liver: a number of studies have shown that it can increase the number of new liver cells to replace old damaged ones.[6] It is used in the treatment of liver disease, and there are now over 450 published papers on its benefits. Milk thistle is one of the oldest herbal remedies, and was used in ancient Rome 'for carrying off bile'.

Because of its powerful antioxidant effects (more powerful than those of either vitamins C or E), milk thistle can help in preventing toxic substances from penetrating liver cells, and minimise the damage done if they do get in.[7]

Milk thistle's positive effect on the liver makes it beneficial for anybody who is working on an alcohol problem. So powerful is its protective action that it can even shield the liver from deathcap mushroom toxins. To put this into perspective, some 30 per cent of people who eat deathcap mushroom will die from poisoning, but milk thistle has a 100 per cent success rate at preventing death from this toxin.[8]

As well being strongly antioxidant, the seeds also contain 60 per cent linoleic acid (see page 61), an essential fatty acid that is extremely important for relieving premenstrual symptoms.

Herbs for depression

St John's wort (*Hypericum perforatum*) has been used for centuries. Along with its well-documented antidepressant effects, St John's wort is also a good remedy for the nervous system and can help to relieve tension and anxiety. It also has diuretic benefits – useful for treating the water retention symptoms of PMS.

St John's wort grows in Europe, Asia and America. It is classed as a weed and has yellow flowers. The small red dots on the petals contain hypericin, a compound that scientists believe is one of the active ingredients responsible for helping depression.

If depression is your main premenstrual symptom, it is worth considering taking St John's wort. Over the past five years interest in this herb as a botanical antidepressant has been enormous. It has been very well researched and a large-scale analysis of twenty-three studies published in the *British Medical Journal* has shown that it is an effective treatment for depression, sleep problems and anxiety.[9]

Because depression is one of the major symptoms of PMS, the benefits of using this herb in this area have begun to attract interest and research. A small trial with nineteen women showed that St John's wort, taken over only two cycles, was helpful both for premenstrual depression and anxiety.[10]

It is thought to work as an antidepressant because it can inhibit the re-uptake of serotonin (see page 42), dopamine and noradrenaline. The pharmaceutical antidepressants that are suggested for PMS are those that stop the re-uptake of serotonin – hence their name, selective serotonin re-uptake inhibitors or SSRIs. St John's wort is effectively working in the same way as a drug, but with fewer side-effects.

It is important to note one side-effect of St John's wort, however. This is increased photosensitivity, particularly in fair-skinned people. What it means in practice is that people who take St John's wort have a greater risk of burning or tanning faster when exposed to the sun. This seems to be particularly problematic if the herb is taken in high doses for long periods of time, but is reversed once taking the herb stopped.

One study compared the effects of St John's wort against the antidepressant imipramine.[11] The results showed that St John's wort was 'therapeutically equivalent' to imipramine – in other words, it worked as well as the antidepressant but, interestingly, was better tolerated. Adverse events were reported in 39 per cent of the participants taking St John's wort, compared to 63 per cent of those taking imipramine. What's more, only 3 per cent of the participants withdrew because of adverse effects from St John's wort compared to 16 per cent taking imipramine.

Note: If you are already taking any medication, such as antidepressants, you need to speak to your doctor before starting St John's wort. It has been suggested that it can stop the Pill from working properly, and there are concerns about interactions with other drugs, such as those for heart problems, blood clots, epilepsy, migraines and immunosuppression after organ transplants, as well as treatments for HIV.

Herbs for stress

The effect of adrenaline on the body has a crucial part to play in controlling premenstrual symptoms, so it is important that you avoid stress wherever possible, and that you ensure that your body is able to cope with, or adapt to, stress in your daily life (see pages 78–86). There is one herb that stands out in its ability to alleviate the effects of stress on the system: Siberian ginseng.

Siberian ginseng (*Eleutherococcus senticosus*)

Siberian ginseng is a shrub that grows in North East Asia. The root of the plant is used for its stress-relieving properties.

This herb is classed as an adaptogen., which means that it works according to your body's needs, providing energy when required, and helping to combat stress and fatigue when you are under pressure. It helps to support adrenal gland function and acts as a tonic to these glands. Siberian ginseng is extremely useful when you have been under mental or physical stress and should be taken for around three months.

It is the most widely researched herb in the world, with over 1,000 scientific studies behind it. As well as having positive effects on the adrenal glands, Siberian ginseng also helps to normalise metabolism and strengthen the immune system. It encourages carbohydrate metabolism and so has a beneficial effect on blood sugar fluctuations, which again helps with premenstrual symptoms – particularly cravings for sugar, chocolate and other foods the week before the period.

Siberian ginseng is not really a true ginseng and should not be confused with panax (Korean) ginseng. Although the latter herb can help with stress, it can also have an overstimulating effect on the body, especially if used with any substances containing caffeine. Research has shown that panax ginseng should not be used by women with fibrocystic breast disease – characterised by lumpy, tender breasts – or for women with an oestrogen-dependent cancer. As PMS is so closely linked to the cycle and fluctuating hormones, it is better to stick to Siberian ginseng alone.

Herbs for cravings

As well as working to balance blood sugar levels (see pages 48–57) through diet and by adding chromium to your supplement programme, you may need a bit of extra help to get any cravings under control in the first few weeks. The easiest way to do this is by using Malabar tamarind.

Malabar tamarind *(Garcinia cambogia)*

The small tropical fruit called the Malabar tamarind is grown in Asia, where the rind is used in Thai and Indian cooking. Garcinia contains HCA (hydroxy-citric acid), which is related to the citric acid found in citrus fruits. HCA encourages your body to use carbohydrates as energy, rather than lay them down as fat. The HCA in this fruit seems to curb appetite and so help reduce food intake, and inhibit the formation of fat and cholesterol.

It may also help to increase the rate at which we burn fat. The theory is that it activates an enzyme called carnitine acetyl-transferase, which speeds up the fat-burning process.[12]

In Chapter 13 you'll find advice on how to put this all together simply. It also gives you information on an excellent product by The Natural Health Practice which contains the most important vitamins, minerals and herbs mentioned above in one pack.

CHAPTER 9

The Treatment Alternatives

As we've seen, diet, lifestyle changes and herbal treatment form the backbone of the natural approach to treating PMS. There are, however, a variety of other therapies and treatments that can encourage the healing process, and ensure that your body is balanced and fighting fit. Not all of these treatments are essential, and you may find that some work better for you than others. They form a complement to the natural treatment of PMS, and work in many different ways to ease symptoms and ensure that your body is working at an optimum level.

Light therapy

Two approaches to light therapy have been used in treating PMS.

The Seasonal Affective Disorder approach

SAD, or Seasonal Affective Disorder, is now a well-known condition – a type of seasonal depression that hits during the dark winter months and lifts during spring and summer. In the winter, the symptoms are very similar to PMS: people not only feel depressed and lethargic, but also crave carbohydrates and sweet foods. So it's not surprising that the light therapy devised to treat SAD can also be used to alleviate PMS.

SAD is believed to stem from an imbalance of melatonin, as well as an increased secretion of cortisol. Both are hormones, the first produced by the pineal gland, the second produced by the adrenals when there is not enough natural light.

In treating SAD, full-spectrum lighting is used to stimulate the pineal gland. Sufferers sit in front of a lamp for a few hours – three is the normal period – at the beginning and end of the day during the winter months. This is not easy to do, and some experts have suggested that sufferers should replace their ordinary lightbulbs with full-spectrum versions so they can have a good blast while they go about their daily life.

To test the theory that PMS could be treated the same way, women with and without PMS were asked to use light therapy over three months, during the week leading up to their period. A dim red light was used as the placebo. It was found that all the light treatments, including the placebo, significantly reduced premenstrual depression.[1] So it is hard to know whether light therapy actually makes a difference. As with most of the PMS trials, the placebo was also beneficial. Furthermore, it would be fairly clear to most women whether or not they were undergoing full-spectrum light treatment, which could, of course, have affected the results.

Photic stimulation

The other kind of light therapy suggested for the treatment of PMS is photic stimulation, or flickering light. With this, a flickering red light is delivered through a mask for about fifteen minutes per day. The theory is that because photic stimulation has been shown previously to induce relaxation[2] and also to help with mood changes, it might have a beneficial effect on PMS symptoms.[3] One study reported in the *Journal of Obstetrics and Gynaecology* found that the PMS symptoms of twelve out of seventeen women improved while they were exposed to the flickering red light every day for up to four cycles.[4] One woman failed to improve and one woman withdrew because her symptoms became worse. The article states that the effects of the light on premenstrual symptoms are greater than the effect of relaxation alone, and suggests that in cases of PMS, the body's external rhythm of day and night may become de-synchronised. The mask is believed to help to re-synchronise the body's clock.

It is impossible to have a placebo group in a trial like this because either the women tested experience the effects of a red flickering light or they don't. This, of course, throws into question the results of the study to some degree. In this particular study, the inventor of the mask was also the main author of the article, so more independent research needs to be done. My question would be, if this is working by re-synchronising the night/day clock, does it stay synchronised in the long term? Or should women continue to use this treatment until the menopause?

The power of the moon

There is also another very interesting aspect of light connected to night and day. It is well known that the effects of day and night can govern an animal's reproductive capabilities. The link seems to be the moon.

As we know, the moon's pull controls the movement of earth's seas. High tides come to that part of the earth closest to the moon.

Every drop of water in the oceans responds to this lunar force and every living marine animal and plant is aware of the rhythm. A certain sea worm swarms to the surface of the sea around the last quarter of the moon. Laboratory experiments have shown that the worm loses its rhythm, swarming at all phases of the moon, if kept under constant light. But if the usual bright light is supplemented on just two nights of the month with another light, the worms swarm exactly one week later. They obviously interpret the extra light as the full moon and act accordingly.

The connection between the moon and the menstrual cycle pops up in many of the world's cultures, and nearly all have a common root word for 'moon' and 'menstruation'. Our own word 'menses' comes from the Latin for 'month', and both are related to the moon. In Africa, the native expression for menstruation is to be 'in the moon'. An average monthly cycle is approximately 28 days, and the lunar cycle is 29.5 days from one full moon to the next.

The melatonin connection

The structure in the body that responds to light is called the pineal gland or pineal body. It is a cone-shaped structure in the brain that secretes the hormone melatonin, which is connected with SAD (see above). Melatonin has a very definite circadian, or daily, rhythm. Its secretion level is ten times higher at night than during the day. Melatonin seems to be the biological timekeeper and it is this internal clock that governs the secretion of different hormones at different times of the day or night. If the pineal gland is damaged or is absent during childhood, children can enter puberty very early. This condition is called 'precocious puberty'. There is, therefore, a very clear link between the pineal gland and reproduction.

It is also known that melatonin inhibits the secretion of luteinising hormone (LH), which is directly linked to ovulation. And we know that in laboratory studies on animals, constant light increases FSH (follicle-stimulating hormone), again linked to ovulation.

When you are trying to eliminate a problem like PMS, which is directly linked to the menstrual cycle, it is worth thinking about something as simple as light. Our bodies are governed by this dark/light cycle at a fundamental level, but our 24-hour society pushes us to override this basic cycle. In fact, with the advent of artificial light, we can turn the whole dark/light cycle upside down. We can go shopping 24 hours a day, eat in the middle of the night when our digestive systems are slowing down, and choose to be exposed to light round the clock, if we so choose.

The other problem with our modern society, certainly in city living, is that even when we go to sleep we are exposed to some light. Street lights, headlights, nightlights, digital clocks and reflections from any form of light are present even in the middle of the night. Light rays can penetrate eyelids, and the dark-adapted retina is very sensitive even to low levels of illumination. The eye sends information about the amounts of light to the pineal gland, which then regulates hormone production accordingly.

It has been suggested that women with PMS and also women with irregular periods should try to eliminate all outside sources of light at night to get the body back to a proper dark/light cycle. This in turn helps to make sure that the pineal gland is functioning correctly, which helps it to orchestrate the correct timing of the secretion of various hormones. It may mean that you need to put up 'black-out' curtains to shut out the street lights, perhaps wear an eye mask to bed, and even change back to a non-digital alarm clock, but the effort may well be worthwhile.

What about supplementing melatonin? In the US, melatonin is sold in supplement form, in much the same way as vitamin C. It has been tested on shift workers to help them synchronise their sleep schedules back again to normal.[5] It has also been recommended for jet lag. Remember, however, that melatonin is a hormone produced by the body, and it should only be taken under the supervision of a medical doctor, and on prescription. There are some cases where melatonin supplementation can be necessary, but only when existing levels are too low.

The aim of natural medicine is to encourage the body to produce the correct amount of hormones at the appropriate times. Adding them as drugs is not the answer, as it does nothing to address the root cause of the problem. The only way to do that is to eat well, get enough sleep, take care of your body through exercise and relaxation, and then to use supplements and herbs to encourage your body to function at optimum level. Short cuts will never achieve long-lasting results, and what this book aims to do is to relieve your symptoms of PMS once and for all.

Psychotherapy

There are hundreds of different approaches in psychotherapy, but one in particular has been very helpful in treating PMS. Cognitive behavioural therapy (CBT) has been used for many other psychological problems, too, including anxiety and depression. For women with PMS, it can be useful as a way of addressing the condition's psychological effects, especially feelings of being 'out of control'.[6] It has been found that the effect of the therapy continues for over four months after sessions have been terminated.

CBT, also known simply as 'cognitive therapy', is based on the understanding that there is a direct relationship between the way we think, feel and behave. Consider the following example: if you repeatedly say to yourself 'Why do I always make mistakes?', your mind affects your behaviour. In other words, you create a self-fulfilling prophecy, which reinforces that negative behaviour.

The aim of cognitive therapy is to help us to overcome problems by changing the way we think. We are taught how to exchange maladjusted thought patterns for more rational thought processes, which, in turn, helps us to gain control over specific situations, behaviours and, ultimately, our lives.

If you do need psychological help, don't hesitate to ask your doctor for a referral (see Useful Addresses on pages 190–1). Because the effect of therapy seems to wear off over time, I would suggest that you undertake both CBT *and* the nutritional approach to treating PMS simultaneously. When you stop attending CBT sessions, your biochemistry will have been fundamentally changed, and the effect will be long-lasting and long-term.

Homeopathy

The word 'homeopathy' comes from the Greek words *omio*, meaning 'same', and *pathos*, meaning 'suffering'. In other words, similar suffering. It reflects the key principle behind the homeopathic method – that a substance can cure the symptoms in an ill person that it is capable of causing in a healthy person.

Every single woman visiting a homeopath will be given a different set of remedies, according to her personal constitution and her unique set of symptoms. Homeopathy is a system of medicine that supports the body's own healing mechanism, using specially prepared remedies. It is 'energy' medicine, in that it works with the body's own energies to encourage healing and to ensure that all body systems are working at optimum level.

Homeopathy is an extremely gentle form of medicine, and it is appropriate and safe for women of all ages, and during pregnancy. The remedy you take contains only the most minute quantities of a substance, so don't panic if you discover you've been prescribed something like belladonna! While some homeopathic remedies can be used at home for 'acute' (short-term) health problems, such as colds and flu, it's essential that you consult a qualified homeopath for anything that you've had for a long time, or that has become recurrent. A homeopath will take a very detailed history that looks at every aspect of you, including your health, symptoms, sleeping patterns, bowel movements, likes and dislikes, emotional factors and much, much more. Remedies are then prescribed, according to your individual requirements.

This individualisation of treatment, which is the cornerstone of natural medicine, means that it is not easy to conduct clinical trials on homeopathy. The double-blind placebo-controlled trial is the 'gold standard' in medicine, but it cannot take into account that we are all unique. In a normal double-blind placebo-controlled trial, to assess, say, the efficacy of a drug for headaches, volunteers would be randomly assigned to either a control group (placebo) or a treatment group (headache drug). The volunteers don't know if they are taking the placebo or the drug, and nor does the scientist running the trial. All of the volunteers in the treatment group get the same dose of headache remedy.

In a trial to show whether homeopathy works for headaches, it would simply not be any good to give the same remedy to the entire treatment group. Homeopathy is prescribed on an individual basis, and what works for one woman will not work for another woman. Their symptoms will differ.

Each person in the treatment group would have to be diagnosed individually and prescribed their own homeopathic remedy. This could still work in the context of a double-blind placebo trial, as long as no one knew whether they were taking a placebo or a remedy.

This individualisation of treatment is much the same with nutrition. Many clinical trials have looked at the effects of particular nutrients (for example, zinc versus a placebo for infertility), but the effects of taking a programme of supplements, designed to treat individual deficiencies, are what needs to be studied against a programme of placebos. But this type of research has simply not been undertaken for nutrition and homeopathy. No account has been taken of the fact that individualisation is the core element of treatment.

With these difficulties in mind, it is not surprising that one double-blind trial studying homeopathic remedies failed to show a benefit for PMS.[7]

There are, however, many homeopathic remedies that are helpful for PMS, and there are many studies in existence showing the efficacy of homeopathy. It can be a process of trial and error to see which one suits you best. Take the remedy twice a day for up to three days, starting one day before your premenstrual symptoms usually begin. If the remedy works and your symptoms disappear, then continue taking the remedy for two or three more days. If it doesn't work, chances are that you need a different remedy. If the symptoms seem worse after taking a homeopathic remedy, this may be a temporary 'healing crisis', which is a sign that your body is working hard to heal itself. Don't panic. Continue taking the remedy and watch to see if the symptoms improve. If they do, you don't need to take the remedy again.

While taking homeopathic remedies, it is best to avoid anything that has a strong smell, such as mint toothpastes, tobacco, coffee, cosmetics and toiletries. Keep the remedies away from any strong-smelling household cleaners, or even aromatherapy oils.

Homeopathic remedies for PMS symptoms

- Nux vomica 30c, if you are craving sweets or fatty foods and are irritable
- Natrum mur 30c, if you are sad and irritable, have fluid retention, swollen breasts and migraines
- Lachesis 30c, for painful breasts and general symptoms of PMS, including headaches
- Pulsatilla 30c, if you are feeling tearful, have painful breasts, and a tendency to irregular periods and nausea
- Sepia 30c, if you crave sweets or salty foods, are tearful, depressed and/or generally feel irritable

Yoga

Yoga classes abound these days, which is lucky: the disclipline has a proven track record in reducing stress and treating PMS. Not only does it offer the same benefits as exercise and relaxation, but it also teaches correct breathing, which can affect overall health. You can practise yoga for as little as five or ten minutes a day and still experience a host of proven benefits.

If you can't get to a yoga class, there are videos available to use at home. Many years ago I learned the Sun Salutation, which is a sequence of yoga positions that flow one into the other. During the sequence you practise deep breathing and spine stretching, and experience improved flexibility, increased circulation and relaxation. The Sun Salutation is illustrated opposite. Strictly speaking, the exercise comprises steps 1 to 4, but I do the whole sequence from 1 to 12, as it exercises both sides of the body. I like to do the entire sequence two or three times.

Reflexology

Reflexology is a gentle therapy that involves stimulating, massaging and applying pressure to points on the hands and feet that correspond to various systems and organs throughout the body, with the aim of stimulating the body's own healing system. These points are called 'reflex points', and each point corresponds to a different body part or function. Reflexology has been shown to be helpful for women with PMS.

In one study, women with PMS were given either 'real' reflexology – in other words, pressure applied to the actual reflex points – or the 'placebo', where pressure was applied to incorrect places. The women getting the 'real' reflexology improved more quickly than the other women.[8] Many women who visit reflexologists report feeling calmer and find it easier to stay in control.

To get the most benefit from reflexology, you'd be best advised to see a registered practitioner whom you can book for regular sessions in the period leading up to menstruation. You can also try it at home. Using the following simple guide, try massaging the relevant points on your feet. Use the edge of your thumb to rub deeply but gently into the appropriate area. Begin sessions the week before your period, and continue once a day during menstruation.

1. Relax both of your feet, and rub the solar plexus point in both feet (in the centre of the foot, beneath the ball of the foot).

2. Using the side of your thumb, rub the area that relates to the pancreas. This is found on the inside edge of the sole of your right foot, and

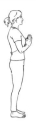 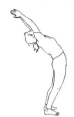 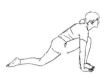

No 1
With your feet together and your arms hanging freely by your sides, stand up straight and hold your shoulders back. Inhale deeply and as you breath out, bring your hands together in front of you.

No 2
Breath in and stretch your arms up high over your head. Lean back from the waist, with your head pushing backwards and your hips pointing forwards

No 3
Breath out and with a slow movement bend forward from the waist. If you can, place your palms flat on the ground on either side of your feet so that there is a straight line across your fingers and toes.

No 4
Breath out and while your hands and feet stay in the same position, push your right leg back and drop your right knee to touch the ground.

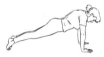 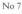 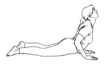 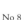 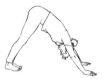

No 5
While holding your breath, stretch your left leg back and keeping both legs straight, hold your body in a diagonal position.

No 6
Breath out, and by bending your knees, rest your knees, forehead and chest on the ground, lifting your buttocks. Your elbows should stay close to the side of your body.

No 7
Breath in and by sliding your hips forward, arch your head and point your toes backwards. Keep your chest up and back and your elbows tucked in close to your side.

No 8
Breath out and keeping your hands in the same position, straighten your arms and push your hips up as high as possible with your feet flat on the ground.

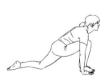 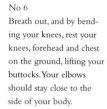 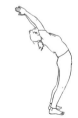 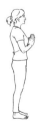

No 9
Breath in and still keeping your hands in the same position, let your hips drop and push your left leg back. Your left knee should now drop to the ground with your arms straight.

No. 10
Breath out and bringing your left leg forward, lift your hips up. If you can, place your palms flat on the ground on either side of your feet so that there is a straight line across your fingers and toes.

No 11
Breath in and stretch your arms up high over your head. Lean back from the waist, with your head pushing backwards and your hips pointing forwards

No 12
With your feet together and your arms hanging freely by your sides, stand up straight and hold your shoulders back. Inhale deeply and as you breath out, bring your hands together in front of you.

Sun Salutation

about halfway down, in the centre of your left sole. This will help to balance blood sugar.

3. The points relating to your kidneys are found about halfway down each sole, in the centre of the foot. Massaging this area can help to stimulate the flow of urine, which can be helpful in periods of fluid retention.

4. Use the top of your thumb to rotate the reflex points for the adrenals. These are found on the inside sole of each foot just above the halfway point, about a centimetre in from the edge of the foot. This action regulates mineral balance, renews energy, and releases a natural form of cortisone, which can help to reduce swelling and inflammation.

5. For headaches and irritability, massage the two big toes, pulling and extending them out.

Sex

It has been suggested that regular sex can help to normalise irregular cycles and reduce PMS symptoms. American reproductive biologist Winnifred Cutler says that the effect is due to male pheromones (smells), which women inhale from their partner when they are naked.[9] Women with short or long cycles took part in the test, and 85 per cent of them returned to a regular 28- to 30-day menstrual cycle after smelling their partner's armpits nightly for three months.

I've not suggested this one to any of my patients yet, but I note that it has to be the same man's armpits that you are sniffing regularly – apparently, multiple pheromones don't have the same normalising effect!

Acupuncture

Acupuncture can be used alongside the other recommendations in this book in order to increase the effectiveness of the treatment. It can also be used alongside conventional treatment. It is a system of Chinese medicine some two millennia old, and is based on the concept of Qi (pronounced *chee*), which is the body's natural energy. An acupuncturist aims to balance the flow of Qi along pathways called meridians. By the insertion of fine needles into the meridians, the body's own healing response can be stimulated. Acupuncture can be particularly useful for correcting hormonal imbalances and generally helping with the symptoms of PMS.

Aromatherapy

This is the use of essential oils which are found in the stem, flowers, leaves, bark, seeds or peel of aromatic plants. Once extracted, these become more concentrated and potent. Each essential oil has its own specific properties and works on two levels: through our sense of smell and by being absorbed via the skin and lungs into the bloodstream, where it has a therapeutic effect on organs, glands and tissue. Except for lavender and tea tree oils, essential oils should be blended in a carrier oil such as almond oil, or diluted in water, before coming into contact with your skin. Drops of essential oil can be used directly in the bath.

Essential oils can be very useful for easing many of the symptoms of PMS, and they can help with problems such as hormonal imbalance, liver problems, stress and poor sleep. Other essential oils such as clary sage are useful for the symptoms of PMS, as they help to lift mood and balance hormones. Fennel can be helpful for water retention and can either be added to the bath or used as a massage oil. Other useful oils include:

- Jasmine, which can help to ease the depression associated with PMS, as well as tension and anxiety
- Juniper, which works on the kidneys and the urinary system, making it an excellent treatment for bloating. It also helps to 'detoxify', and to support the action of the liver.
- Grapefruit oil, which works mainly on the liver and gall bladder, so can be useful for constipation, headaches and liverish complaints, all of which can affect PMS
- Geranium, which has a cooling, regulating effect and can help with conditions affecting the nervous system as well as restlessness and anxiety
- Rosemary, which can help to prevent fluid retention when used in regular massage
- Bergamot and chamomile, which are effective in reducing depression and irritability

• Lavender, which can help to reduce tension and encourage balance and a good healthy sleep

Some oils are not appropriate for pregnancy. Check with a qualified practitioner before using any oil in pregnancy.

Massage

One of the oldest, simplest forms of therapy, massage is a system of stroking, pressing and kneading different areas of the body to relieve pain, relax, stimulate and tone. Massage does much more than make you feel good (although it helps with that!). It also works on soft tissues (muscles, tendons and ligaments) to improve muscle tone. Although it largely affects muscles just under the skin, it is believed that it also reaches the deeper layers of muscles and possibly even the organs themselves. Massage also stimulates blood circulation and assists the lymphatic system, which runs parallel to the circulatory system, improving elimination of toxic waste throughout the body.

There are many more therapies widely used in the treatment of women's health conditions and as each woman is an individual, it is worthwhile experimenting and finding those that suit you best.

CHAPTER 10

Coping with the Symptoms

Let's say you're following the dietary recommendations in Chapter 5, and have embarked on your three-month regime of regularly taking the right nutritional supplements and herbs. Soon your body will reach a state of good health, and your PMS symptoms will disappear. So far, so good. But the long-term aim of this programme is to eliminate PMS completely. And you may find that as your body becomes healthier and more balanced, you still continue to experience some symptoms that affect the quality of your life. In this situation, the following recommendations will help to ease symptoms while your body recovers.

The symptoms I discuss below are the ones most women describe as being the most common and uncomfortable.

Sugar and food cravings

Up to 60 per cent of women experience sugar cravings in the week leading up to their period. Many women have admitted that they are capable of eating whole boxes of chocolates or packets of biscuits during the premenstrual period, while these same foods do not hold anywhere near the same appeal in the remainder of their cycle.

Some women crave foods other than sweets, and feel the need to gorge themselves for inexplicable reasons. Alcohol can be a particular problem during this time, partly because some women feel more stressed and in need of instant relaxation, and also because it lifts blood sugar levels in the short term. Women can become more sensitive to alcohol premenstrually, which means they get drunk more easily and cannot tolerate it in the way that they usually can.

This effect has never been fully explained, but it is interesting that this intolerance to alcohol is also seen in people who have candida (a yeast overgrowth – see pages 154–9). Women with candida find that they feel drunk on a small amount of alcohol, and research has shown that for women who have tried 'everything' to get rid of their PMS symptoms, relief came only when they were treated for candida.[1]

These food and alcohol cravings cannot be 'controlled' psychologically. In other words, telling yourself to exert some self-control and avoid problem foods simply won't work. All of us experience times when we eat too much, and under normal circumstances self-restraint is the key. However, during the premenstrual period, the cravings we experience are biochemical urges, where our bodies are actually demanding a certain type of food to fulfil a genuine need. The body seems to be trying to prevent or correct a too-sudden or prolonged drop in blood sugar, which in turn would cause adrenaline to be released, thereby blocking the uptake of the hormone progesterone.

So why doesn't this happen every day of the month? It seems that the interaction between the fluctuating female hormones and fluctuating blood sugar levels causes the cravings to become more extreme.

The best and, really, the only way to control sugar or food cravings is to make sure that you are eating little and often. As explained in Chapter 5, eating regularly will help to keep your blood sugar in balance. If your blood sugar drops (causing hypoglycaemia, or low blood sugar) your body will demand that you sort it out immediately. The easy way to get this 'quick fix' is to put more sugar into your system, which will give a fast and high rise in blood sugar.

Your blood sugar reaches this low point if you go too long without eating (over three hours in the premenstrual period), or when your diet is based mainly around foods containing sugar and caffeine. These foods provide a quick blood sugar 'high', leading to as quick a slump. This type of diet creates a self-perpetuating vicious circle, where you need the food for its effects on your blood sugar, but find it actually makes the situation worse – so you need another quick fix to balance it out again.

In order to prevent the cravings, you have the break this cycle. The easiest way to do this is to eliminate caffeine and sugar, while eating good-quality carbohydrates (see pages 50–1) on a 'little and often' basis. This will prevent your blood sugar from surging and dropping, and without these dips, you will find that your cravings are under control.

Natural remedies

As well as making sure that you eat little and often to eliminate the cravings, you can, for a short period of, say, three months, use some natural nutrients and remedies to help this process.

The most important ones for sugar and food cravings are chromium, the herb *Garcinia cambogia* and several homeopathic remedies.

Chromium is especially important in controlling sugar and food cravings because it is an essential mineral for the metabolism of sugar. Without it, insulin is less effective in controlling blood sugar levels. Chromium also helps to reduce hunger, which can be helpful for those women who have premenstrual surges in appetite and crave any food.

Take the programme of supplements outlined on pages 173–4 and make sure that you are getting a total of 200mcg of chromium from them. You may need to add in extra chromium if you experience food and sugar cravings, as there will probably not be enough in your multivitamin and mineral supplement.

> **Warning:** If you are diabetic, you need to speak to your doctor before supplementing with chromium.

Garcinia cambogia (see page 117) is a small tropical fruit called the Malabar tamarind, which contains HCA (hydroxy-citric acid). The HCA in this fruit helps to curb the appetite and can be used beneficially while you are working on your diet. The HCA also helps your body to use carbohydrates as energy, rather than laying them down as fat.

Some supplement companies sell a combination of chromium and *Garcinia cambogia,* but do not take the Garcinia if you are prone to migraines.

Two homeopathic remedies (see pages 123–5) are indicated for food and sugar cravings:

- Sepia 30c, if you crave sweet or salty foods
- Nux vomica 30c, if you crave sweet or fatty foods.

There are a number of other appropriate remedies, but they will work best if they are prescribed by a homeopath according to your specific symptoms.

Water retention

As we've seen, this is a problem for many women and it is often worse just before a period. Don't be tempted to limit your intake of fluids – this can actually cause bloating, as your body will think it needs to conserve water. Water is a natural diuretic and it should be drunk as frequently as possible, particularly when you are retaining water.

Cut down on your intake of salt, which can encourage water retention (see pages 68–9). Table salt is sodium chloride, and sodium is a mineral that affects your body's ability to balance water retention and blood pressure. Another mineral, potassium, works with sodium to regulate water balance and normalise heart rhythm. The more sodium you consume, the more potassium you need to counteract this effect. The World Health Organization recommends a maximum of 6g (1 rounded teaspoon) of salt a day. This supplies us with 2,400mg of sodium. We only need 500mg of sodium a day to stay healthy.

Sodium is found naturally in all fruits, vegetables and grains, and is already present in most ready-prepared foods, including salad dressing, biscuits, bread, sauces and even tinned vegetables. Most people end up eating about 9g of salt a day and it is all too easy to consume too much without realising it. One burger in a bun can contain 6g, two slices of wholemeal bread 1.2g and a slice of cheese and tomato pizza 5.3g. Two slices of bread contain more salt than a packet of crisps.

We also consume sodium as sodium nitrate, which is the preservative used in meat, and as monosodium glutamate, the flavour enhancer used extensively in convenience and Chinese food.

If you have a high salt intake, you could be carrying around an extra 1.8kg (4lb) in excess weight due to water retention. A 1998 government report on nutrition and heart disease by the Committee on Medical Aspects concluded that the reduction of salt in the diet by a third could save at least 34,000 lives a year. The usual first-line treatment for high blood pressure is diuretics, which work by preventing the reabsorption of sodium and potassium. Doctors also recommend that we reduce our salt intake, lose weight, take regular exercise, cut down on alcohol and stop smoking.

Water retention can also be caused by the same blood sugar swings that trigger many premenstrual symptoms.

When blood sugar drops, adrenaline is automatically released into the bloodstream to move sugar from our cells into the blood to try to rectify this imbalance. At the same time, when the sugar leaves the cells it is replaced by water, which causes the puffiness and bloating associated with water retention. So by following the recommendations on pages 48–57 to get your blood sugar in balance you will also help to reduce water retention.

Many women who suffer from water retention turn to diuretics. These will certainly increase the rate at which fluid is lost, but important minerals will also be flushed from your body, including, as I have mentioned, potassium, which is crucial for heart function.

Natural remedies

Dandelion (see pages 113–14) is a natural herbal diuretic that allows fluid to be released without the loss of vital nutrients. It contains more vitamins and minerals than any other herb and is one of the best natural sources of potassium.

Parsley is also a useful diuretic and can simply be eaten as part of your diet. Initially, however, if you are suffering from extreme water retention, it would be worth taking it in tincture form for a couple of months. It could be mixed with dandelion to give a combination tincture.

Homeopathic remedies can also be useful for water retention and the remedy most specifically indicated for this is Natrum mur, especially if you also feel sad and irritable in the time leading up to your period.

Aromatherapy oils can be very effective in countering water retention. Fennel, which acts to detoxify and is particularly indicated for any 'swollen' or 'bloated' conditions, can be added to a warm bath (approximately ten drops). Soak for about fifteen to twenty minutes for best effect. Juniper also helps with bloating and puffiness and can be either added to a bath or used in a massage oil.

Headaches and migraines

Headaches are one of the most common premenstrual symptoms. Some women only suffer headaches or migraine attacks just before or on the first day of their period. About 6 million people in Britain suffer migraines, but women sufferers outnumber men by three to one.

Headaches and migraines are different. Headaches are painful but are not usually accompanied by other symptoms. Migraines usually follow a pattern of symptoms and these can be different for each individual. Some sufferers experience warning symptoms (known as an 'aura') before the pain starts, and these can include blurring and changes in vision, yawning and fatigue and numbness on one side of the body. The pain itself can be accompanied by nausea and sometimes vomiting. Migraines occur when the blood vessels in the brain alternately constrict and then dilate.

During migraines, before the changes in blood vessels there is also a change in brain chemistry. Serotonin is released, affecting the hypothalamus in the brain. The serotonin swells the blood vessels in the brain. These engorged vessels irritate and inflame the nerves. This stimulates the vessels to swell further, causing a cycle of pain which can last for hours or even days. Prostaglandins can also be stimulated and if there is an increase in the production of PGE2, or 'bad', prostaglandins (see pages 61–2), this can increase the inflammatory response and pain.

There are different types of headaches. One of the most common forms of headache is known as a tension headache. Given that PMS was initially known as premenstrual *tension* or PMT, it is easy to see why the premenstrual time of the month can herald tension headaches. This type of headaches can feel like a band around the head, and extend down into the neck and shoulder muscles.

Another headache associated with PMS is known as a sinus headache, caused by swelling of the cells at the entrance to the sinus. This is actually another sign of water retention, which is a common feature of PMS for many women.

Nobody knows the cause of premenstrual headaches and migraines but it is suggested that they are triggered by low levels of oestrogen before menstruation. Other suggestions are that fluctuating hormones just before the period make us more sensitive to the usual headache or migraine triggers. Some 80 per cent of migraine sufferers stop having headaches when they become pregnant, so there is an obvious correlation there. The contraceptive Pill can also trigger migraines.

Whatever the pattern of your headaches, follow all of the dietary recommendations noted in Chapter 5, and pay particular attention to the section on blood sugar. Missing meals or eating irregularly can actually trigger a headache or migraine at any time, but especially so premenstrually, when you will be more sensitive to those fluctuations.

Natural remedies

Magnesium is a muscle relaxant, and a deficiency in this mineral can cause blood vessels to go into spasm. Ensuring that you have enough magnesium is extremely important in preventing premenstrual headaches and migraine attacks. Taking magnesium every day has been shown to help not only the intensity but also the duration of the migraines, as compared to placebos.[2] Take 250 to 350mg twice a day, every day of the month.

Include good amounts of both omega 3 and omega 6 essential fatty acids (see page 61) in order to keep the 'bad' prostaglandins under control. One study showed that migraine sufferers experienced a significant reduction in both the frequency and the intensity of the attack by taking omega 3 fish oils every day.[3]

The herb feverfew (*Tanacetum parthenium*) can also be a good treatment for migraines and headaches. The active ingredient in feverfew is partheniolide, which helps to dilate blood vessels. Feverfew also blocks the production of the inflammatory prostaglandin PGE2. Use tea, tincture or extract with 250mcg of partheniolide and take three times daily. Seventy per cent of migraine sufferers in one study found that their attacks occurred less frequently, or were prevented altogether, by taking feverfew.[4]

Use herbs such as milk thistle (see pages 114–15) to improve liver function. The more effectively your liver is working, the better it will be able to deal with fluctuating hormones leading up to your period. A healthy liver will also be able to produce all of the enzymes needed to break down certain foods that might trigger a migraine.

It is also possible to suffer pain as a result of taking too many painkillers. This can become a vicious circle, as many over-the-counter painkillers contain codeine or caffeine, which makes them addictive. It is also possible to develop an intolerance to painkillers so that the dosage has to be increased to get an effect, which leads to a rebound headache and a need for more painkillers.

Aromatherapy and homeopathy may also help you cope with premenstrual headaches.

Food triggers

When you get a headache or migraine, make a note of what occurred on that day. Write down what you ate, what time you ate, and consider the sort of day you were having. Were you feeling stressed, overworked or just tired? See if you can find a pattern or a trigger. If you only get a migraine once a month, it is possible to have a food trigger to which you are only sensitive premenstrually, when your hormones are fluctuating. But if you suffer from migraines throughout your cycle, you may have a food trigger that affects you at all times of the month, perhaps more pronounced before your period.

Certain foods contain substances, such as tyramine, phenylethylamine and histamine, that trigger migraines in susceptible women. The foods containing them can include cheese, citrus fruits, red wine, chocolate and coffee. There will be a time lag between eating the food and suffering an attack, which is why it is not always easy to spot the food causing a problem. The time lag is due to the fact that the problem arises when the food reaches the liver, and should be broken down by enzymes.

For instance, red wine can be a problem, as it contains high levels of chemicals known as phenols. Usually an enzyme destroys these chemicals, but migraine sufferers seem to have low levels of this enzyme, and the red wine seems to inhibit the enzyme even further. Without these enzymes, substances called vasodilating amines are released, which expand the blood vessels of the brain. Some foods contain a number of substances that can cause a problem. Both alcohol and chocolate contain phenylethylamine, for example, and cheese contains tyramine. The same foods can also contain histamine or histamine-releasing compounds. For instance, red wine contains 20 to 200 times more histamine than white wine.

Foods that contain these dietary amines (histamine, tyramine, phenylethylamine and so on) can trigger a migraine by causing blood vessels to expand in those who are sensitive to these substances.[5]

You may be able to work out your own triggers. However, if you can't find a link, a simple blood test can assess this for you. You need to be careful about the kind of blood test you choose because a normal food allergy test will measure antibodies, which are triggered by the immune system. With migraines, the problem is not triggered by the immune system but by chemicals within the foods. I have described a blood test appropriate for migraines on page 175.

Tips for easing a headache

These tips are designed to help while you are having an attack, but the main aim is to put the dietary, supplement and herbal recommendations into place. These will, ultimately, prevent your headaches from occurring.

1. Massage

Rubbing the temples can help to relieve the pain. A neck and shoulder massage should also help. Using a blend of relaxing, analgesic essential oils (see pages 129–30) can give an extra boost.

2. Hot and cold

Putting an ice pack on the area where the pain is centred can reduce the blood flow, which allows the muscles to relax. However, it has been found that the side of the head affected by the pain seems to be cooler than the other. In this instance, heat may be more useful. You'll need to experiment with each of these, to discover which is more useful for your individual symptoms.

Some migraine sufferers actually feel better after having a warm bath, especially if an essential oil such as lavender is added, while others find that putting their feet in warm water is effective.

3. Muscle relaxation exercise

To help relax the muscles, particularly when you have a tension headache, sit in a chair and place your elbows on a table. Clasp your hands together round the back of your head and slowly press your chin down on your chest. Hold this position for two minutes. Use your hands to turn your head to the right. Hold for two minutes and then come back to the centre. Use your hands to turn your head to the left and hold again for two minutes before releasing.

4. Acupuncture

Acupuncture can be an extremely useful treatment for headaches and migraines and could be used alongside the dietary and supplement approach.

5. Orgasm

Some women find that having an orgasm can help get rid of a headache, as it helps to open up the blood vessels. Other women, however, find that sex can actually bring on a headache. There is a condition called benign orgasmic cephalgi, which is a sharp one-sided headache experienced during sex. These coital headaches do not occur every time and will go away by themselves within minutes or, at most, a few hours.

6. Homeopathy

A homeopath will look at your constitution and lifestyle and prescribe an individual remedy (see pages 123–4) according to your specific symptoms. There are, however, some good remedies for treating acute headaches:

• Natrum muriaticum (Natrum mur). This is the main remedy when the headaches are period-related. It's particularly useful if your symptoms include fluid retention, swollen breasts, and feeling sad and irritable.

- Lycopodium. This remedy is appropriate when the pain is right-sided and connected with missing meals.
- Spigelia is useful when the pain is left-sided and associated with pressure on the eye.
- Belladonna is one of the best remedies for headaches, particularly when there is throbbing. It's indicated for many types of migraine, and headaches associated with a flushed face and dilated pupils.
- Aconite is for headaches that come on suddenly, feel worse in the cold or in a draught, and are experienced like a tight band around the head. It's indicated if you feel apprehensive.
- For bursting, aching headaches, a hypersensitive scalp and symptoms that are worse in damp, foggy weather, try Hypericum.
- For headaches associated with irritability, which are worse first thing in the morning and feel like a dizzy, dull bruising pain, try Nux vomica. It's also helpful for headaches caused by overindulgence in foods and alcohol, which is common during the premenstrual period.
- Bryonia will help if your head feels bruised, and there are sharp, stabbing pains that are made worse by moving your eyes.
- Pulsatilla helps when you feel tearful, miserable and generally headachy.

7. Aromatherapy

Both lavender and chamomile can quell a headache, especially if used at the immediate onset of pain. Other useful oils include rosemary, which can stimulate the blood supply to the head, and eucalyptus, which eases pain and reduces any congestion. Add a few drops of one to a warm bath, or make up a massage oil to apply as a neck and shoulder massage.

Breast tenderness

Up to 70 per cent of women in the West experience breast changes that fluctuate with their menstrual cycles. The breasts can feel so tender, swollen and/or lumpy that the discomfort is unbearable. Some women complain that they can't bear to be hugged, and find sleeping very difficult because they can't get comfortable.

There are a number of medical terms used to describe these breast changes and they can include cyclical breast pain or mastalgia, cyclical mastitis or fibrocystic breast disease. Despite their severity and the disruption they can cause, most breast problems are benign, and not related to cancer. However, don't be tempted to ignore them. Any unusual changes in your breasts should be reported to your doctor.

Because the symptoms are linked to the cycle, it could be easy to say that breast tenderness and lumpiness are 'caused' by the hormone changes in the cycle. But it is interesting to note that women who live in Asian countries like Japan don't experience the same degree of breast changes, although they have the same hormones circulating each month.[6] What's the main difference between Eastern and Western women? Apart from geography, it's largely diet. That's why what you eat is so important in controlling any of the symptoms of PMS.

If breast tenderness is your main premenstrual symptom, you should avoid any drinks or foods that normally contain caffeine. In these foods are a family of substances called methylxanthines which includes not only caffeine but also theophylline and theobromine. These methylxanthines, which have been proven to increase problems with painful, lumpy and tender breasts, known as fibrocystic breast disease, are found in coffee, black tea, green tea, chocolate, cola and even decaffeinated coffee, as well as in medications that contain caffeine, such as headache remedies.

A link has also been found between fibrocystic breast disease and constipation. One study showed that women who had fewer than three bowel movements per week had a 4.5 times greater chance of having breast problems than women who had a bowel movement every day.[8] It is important that you have an adequate intake of fibre in the form of whole grains, vegetables and fruits to ensure regularity. Don't be tempted to take bran, which can add to the problem and irritate your gut. Bran contains substances called phytates, which can block the uptake of valuable minerals such as iron, calcium and magnesium. As a magnesium deficiency is quite common in PMS, you don't want to be exacerbate the situation by preventing your body from absorbing the magnesium found in food.

If you need extra help, sprinkle 15ml (1 tablespoon) of linseeds – also known as flaxseeds – on to your breakfast cereal in the morning, or soak 15ml (1 tablespoon) of linseeds in a small amount of water and then swallow. Ensure that you are drinking plenty of fresh water, particularly if you are taking linseeds.

Make sure that you are eating well and following the dietary recommendations in Chapter 5. Also include good amounts of phytoestrogens (see pages 66–8) as these weak, naturally occurring oestrogens can help to keep any excesses of hormones in check and may explain why the majority of Asian women do not experience breast discomfort as we do. Phytoestrogens are effectively 'plant' oestrogens, and they are found in foods such as soya, chickpeas and lentils. Include them all in your diet as often as you can.

Natural remedies

You may need to add some extra nutrients for about three months if breast tenderness is a major problem for you. If you are sensitive to the methylxanthines in coffee and chocolate, it may not take as long as three months to resolve. Simply cutting out foods with caffeine can and will make a dramatic difference to your symptoms.

Iron, in the form of the inorganic iron ferrous sulphate, can also give you constipation which can increase breast tenderness. For one thing, you should really only be taking iron if you have a deficiency. If a blood test shows that iron supplements are necessary because you are anaemic, and you suffer from constipation as a result, you should change to an organic form of iron which does not have the same side-effects.

Vitamin E has been shown to help reduce breast pain and tenderness in a number of studies and is worth supplementing over a couple of months to see if it helps ease your symptoms.[9]

Cyclical breast changes may be due to an excess of oestrogen over progesterone. Lactobacillus acidophilus (see page 70) helps to increase the levels of enzymes that work to reabsorb the 'old' oestrogens in your body. These probiotics (beneficial bacteria) also help to improve the transit time of a bowel movement. The longer waste material stays in your system, the more 'old' hormones and toxins can be reabsorbed back into your body.

As mentioned on page 100, the B vitamins are important generally for eliminating PMS, but they are of particular value if you suffer from breast discomfort. The B vitamins will help your liver break down 'old' oestrogens that can be playing havoc with your cycle and creating an excess of oestrogen because 'old' hormones are not being eliminated properly. Taking a B-complex supplement can help to reduce breast symptoms for this reason.

Essential fatty acids are an important part of a healthy diet, but research has shown that supplementing with evening primrose oil which contains GLA (gamma-linolenic acid) can have a significantly positive effect on breast discomfort.[10] The GLA helps to control the production of a 'bad' prostaglandin called PGE2, which can cause heat and inflammation in the breasts if levels are too high. GLA also increases the level of another 'good' prostaglandin, PGE1, which can help to balance the effect of prolactin on the breasts.

Research has also shown that evening primrose oil may be most helpful to women whose main premenstrual symptoms is breast tenderness or fibrocystic breast disease (which is a cyclical condition as well).[11] It usually needs to be taken for about three months to be effective, so don't give up.

It is now possible to get evening primrose oil on prescription in the UK. The GLA content is normally 40mg per capsule, and you may need to take up to eight capsules a day to achieve the desired effect (the suggested dosage is between 240 and 320mg per day). The GLA content in each capsule varies tremendously among supplement producers, so it's worth scouting around for a brand with higher levels of GLA.

Evening primrose oil is only one of the important oils studied for its effect on breast discomfort. Oils from starflower, blackcurrant seed and borage may be just as effective.

> **Warning:** Check with your doctor before taking any capsules containing GLA if you have a history of epilepsy.

The omega 3 fatty acids are especially important for healthy breasts because they have been shown to inhibit tumour growth. Many studies have shown that the omega-3 fatty acids have a protective role to play in breast cancer.[12]

Take the herb agnus-castus (see pages 111–12), which helps to balance the hormones. Also take milk thistle (see pages 114–15) to ensure that your liver processes oestrogen efficiently, allowing any excess to be properly excreted. The herb *Ginkgo biloba* has also proved useful, and a trial conducted by a hospital in France has shown that women who took ginkgo had significantly less premenstrual breast pain than those who took a placebo.[13] Ginkgo helps to increase circulation and can also reduce swelling.

There are a number of essential oils that can be useful. You can blend them together and massage them into your breasts, or use a few drops in your bath. For example, fennel, geranium, juniper and lavender can help to encourage lymph drainage and help to regulate hormone imbalances, thereby relieving breast pain.

Similarly, homeopathic remedies, taken from about a day or so before your symptoms normally begin, may help. The best ones to try are:

- Lachesis, for painful breasts, and symptoms that are worse in the morning

- Calcarea, when your breasts are painful and swollen, you crave eggs and sweet things, and feel tired and lacking energy
- Pulsatilla, for painful breasts, and feeling sick and tearful
- Natrum mur, which is excellent for fluid retention, swollen breasts, and feeling sad and irritable

Mood swings

Is one of your main symptoms extreme personality changes, where you just don't feel the same person in the second half of the month? Do you get irritable, angry, depressed, tearful and/or anxious? It is interesting that women describe being totally aware of what is happening – being irritable with the children, getting angry with their partners, crying for no particular reason, feeling very sad, flying off the handle and becoming irrational at any insignificant thing – and yet, are not able to control it. Once their period arrives, they feel like a different person. It's easy to rationalise that it won't happen again the next month, but, inevitably, the same symptoms recur and most women are powerless to stop it.

If this situation sounds familiar, it is extremely important that you put into place the blood sugar recommendations straight away (see pages 48–57). These symptoms are classic signs that your blood sugar has dropped and that adrenaline has been released. What you are experiencing is the effect of an adrenaline surge. You are all geared up for 'fight or flight', except most of it comes out as fight!

It would be interesting to look at when you get these outbursts. They will often happen if you have missed a meal or you have to wait to eat until your partner comes home. Most women feed their children and then wait to eat with their partners. If they haven't had much lunch, their bodies are forced to go a very long time without much food, causing a major dip in blood sugar levels. Not surprisingly, everything explodes when their partner comes in.

Make sure you are eating little and often, and eliminate anything with caffeine or sugar, which increases the roller-coaster of blood sugar swings.

Natural remedies

Definitely include a B-complex supplement in addition to your usual multivitamin and mineral tablet. The B vitamins are known as the 'stress' vitamins. B6 is especially important because it is needed to make serotonin, the 'antidepressant' neurotransmitter. Also include magnesium, known as 'nature's tranquilliser', and some essential fatty acids (see pages 63–4) such as linseed oil capsules.

Along with the combination of herbs mentioned on page 174, make sure that you add in Siberian ginseng to help adrenal function, because it's likely that you have depleted adrenal function due to continual adrenaline surges.

Essential oils can be very effective, blended and used in a massage or added to the bath. Try lavender, which is calming and relaxing. Bergamot, chamomile and rose oils are effective in reducing depression and irritability, while clary sage, sandalwood and ylang ylang are oils that are both sedative and antidepressant.

There are huge numbers of homeopathic remedies that are appropriate, including the following:

- Pulsatilla when you are tearful and sad for no reason
- Lycopodium, when you are feeling bad-tempered and depressed
- Causticum, when you are feeling pessimistic, irritable and over-sensitive, with a frequent urge to urinate
- Sepia when you are feeling irritable, chilly, weepy and emotionally flat, and perhaps also crave sweet or salty foods
- Nux vomica, when you feel irritable and chilly, with constipation, frequent urination and cravings for sweet or fatty foods

Lack of co-ordination/clumsiness

It is well known that women can be more accident-prone in the week or so leading up to their period.[14] It seems that the nervous system is affected, giving rise to a lack of co-ordination and often clumsiness. Many women are aware that their driving is affected premenstrually, and I have seen a number of women who actually avoid driving in the week before their periods. This is not always practical! The aim here is to get rid of the problem.

Your nervous system is a vast network of cells that carry information in the form of nerve impulses in order to bring about activity in your body. Your brain and spinal cord together form the central nervous system and the other nervous tissue is known as the autonomic nervous system, which brings about changes in bodily function that you can't consciously control, such as heartbeat, sweating, and immune activity. The autonomic nervous system is then split into the sympathetic and parasympathetic nervous systems.

When you are stressed, the sympathetic nervous system is dominant and releases adrenaline. It is basic to the fight-or-flight mechanism and increases the general level of activity in the body. The parasympathetic nervous system governs the relaxation response and is involved in the repair and maintenance of our bodies. It also controls the digestive system. The parasympathetic nervous system releases a neurotransmitter called acetylcholine.

There is a delicate balance between the two parts of your autonomic nervous system, and it is not known exactly how premenstrual changes affect them. We do know, however, that adrenaline plays a major part in PMS and this may be upsetting the delicate balance.

Many of the actions we adopt to avoid accidents are instinctive and require us to respond rapidly without time to think. While driving we can sometimes be aware that we have driven from A to B safely without even consciously thinking about what we were doing because our mind was on something else. And yet if a child had run into the road, then instinctively we would have swerved or braked instantly to avoid an accident. It may be that delicate changes in the nervous system during the premenstrual time delay this type of reaction.

Follow all the dietary recommendations in Chapter 5, focusing in particular on eating little and often, and cutting out caffeine and sugar. This will ensure that adrenaline is not being released inappropriately, and that your sympathetic nervous system is not working overtime.

Learn a relaxation technique such as progressive relaxation (see pages 83–4) so that the parasympathetic nervous system becomes dominant and your body has extra time for repair and maintenance. Just five to ten minutes a day can be enough.

Natural remedies

Make sure that you are taking a B-complex tablet alongside your multi-vitamin and mineral supplement. Although you need a good supply of all of the B vitamins, the most important of these is vitamin B5, called pantothenic acid. B5 is needed to make the neurotransmitter acetylcholine, which is released by the parasympathetic nervous system. Vitamin B5 is found in whole grains, like brown rice, wholemeal bread, legumes, cauliflower, salmon, broccoli, tomatoes and sweet potatoes. If lack of co-ordination or clumsiness is a problem, just make sure you add in a sepa-rate B5 on top of the multivitamin and mineral mentioned on page 108, so that you are getting 50mg of vitamin B5 per day (including the B5 in your multivitamin and mineral tablet).

Also include magnesium and Siberian ginseng, which can help to control the stress response. You could also take the herb ginkgo, which has beneficial effects on the nervous system. It is thought that it helps to deliver oxygen and blood sugar to nerve cells. Include 200mg of magnesium a day and use the Siberian ginseng and ginkgo as tinctures over a period of three months.

Relaxing and rejuvenating essential oils may be useful, including lavender, chamomile and melissa, which is soothing to both the mind and the body. Melissa also has a calming and regulating effect on the menstrual cycle, which can help to ease problems that may be causing the clumsiness. Homeopathic remedies are also helpful. Try one of the following:

- Causticum, when you are oversensitive and inclined to burst into tears
- Lycopodium, if you lack self-confidence and feel poorly co-ordinated during the premenstrual period
- Other useful remedies such as Sepia, Pulsatilla and Natrum mur

Lack of concentration/memory

A number of women say that they find it hard to concentrate premenstru-ally, and struggle to remember things that they would normally find easy. You may need to read and reread a page of a book or an article, for exam-ple, because you simply haven't taken in anything while reading the first time, or you may find yourself daydreaming, when you are normally a very focused person.

This inability to concentrate and changes in memory are part and parcel of the symptoms of PMS. As you change your eating habits, and begin to eat regularly, taking the recommended supplements, these symptoms will start to disappear.

Natural remedies

You can also help aid this process by adding in the herb *Gingko biloba*, which has been found to have a rejuvenating effect on the brain. A number of clinical trials have shown that it improves learning ability, memory and concentration.

Ginkgo helps to deliver oxygen and encourages blood supply to the brain. Our brain's 'food' is oxygen, so if the blood supply to the brain is insufficient, our mental function can be impaired. Brain cells alone account for 25 per cent of the body's total oxygen consumption. A study in the *Lancet* found that *Ginkgo biloba* could improve blood flow to the head, increase the supply of glucose and oxygen, which the brain needs to create energy, prevent blood clots and protect the brain cells against damage.[15]

Skin problems

Acne, spots, greasy skin, skin eruptions such as boils – these are just a few of the skin changes women can experience in the lead-up to their periods.

There are three major forms of acne. Acne conglobata is the most severe form, in which cysts form underneath the skin; these can become infected and cause scarring. Acne rosacea occurs when the nose and cheeks are very red and often covered with spots. Acne vulgaris is the least severe form of acne and is connected to changes in the oil-secreting glands of the skin. This type of acne usually varies with the cycle, and is the one most commonly related to PMS.

Acne is very common around puberty and often affects boys more than girls. It is caused by blockages in the sebaceous glands which are responsible for producing a waterproofing substance called sebum. The sebum is a mixture of oils and waxes that lubricates the skin. If this mix is too thick, the pores become blocked as the sebum is excreted through the pores of the skin, causing acne.

Testosterone increases the production of sebum, hence the fact that boys at puberty are affected more than girls. But women also produce androgens (male hormones) from the ovaries and from the adrenal glands. Recent research has shown that two-thirds of women who have acne have raised levels of androgens[16] so there is a definite hormone imbalance. There is a condition called polycystic ovary syndrome (PCOS), characterised by acne, weight gain and excess hair and caused by hormonal imbalances, usually with high androgen levels. If you have these symptoms, you should see your doctor for a check-up. For more information on PCOS, see my book *Nutritional Health Handbook for Women*.

In women who get acne only in the premenstrual period, it has been suggested that the adrenal glands are producing too much of these androgens just before a period. Furthermore, oestrogen helps to regulate the production of sebum, but in the days before a period, oestrogen levels fall. Therefore, more sebum can be produced, blocking the pores.

Because the adrenal glands play a part in premenstrual acne, it is crucial that you're following all of the recommendations for regulating blood sugar and controlling stress to ensure that the adrenal glands are functioning healthily. The other reason why it is so important to get your blood sugar in balance if you have premenstrual acne is that excess circulating insulin will stimulate the ovaries to produce more testosterone and more sebum, which results in blocked pores.

As well as eating little and often and eliminating those foods and drinks that can upset the sugar balance, include more phytoestrogens (see pages 66–8) in your diet. Phytoestrogens help your body to stimulate the production of sex hormone-binding globulin, or SHBG,[17] which is a protein produced by the liver that binds sex hormones, such as testosterone, in order to control how much is circulating in the blood at any one time.

The usual treatment for acne is antibiotics, but this is not recommended in the case of PMS. It does nothing to address the real cause of the problem which is, of course, related to your cycle. Furthermore, the use of antibiotics is likely to increase the overgrowth of candida (see pages 154–9).

Natural remedies

If you have been told that you have high testosterone levels, follow all of the other recommendations below for skin problems. Also add in a herb called saw palmetto (*Serenoa repens*). It comes from a small palm tree found in North America, whose berries are used in tinctures or capsule form.

Research has shown that saw palmetto works as an anti-androgen, which can be very helpful for premenstrual acne.[18]

It can be taken either as a tincture (1 teaspoon three times a day), added to the other balancing herbs on page 174, or as a supplement containing 320mg of standardised extract a day.

Also while you are working on balancing your blood sugar, make sure that your supplement programme (see pages 173–4) gives you 200mcg of chromium in total a day – or add in extra chromium to top it up to 200mcg.

Vitamin B6 has been shown to be beneficial for premenstrual acne.[19] Ensure that you are getting 50mg of vitamin B6 in total per day.

With other skin problems that appear premenstrually, it is important to make sure that you are eating as healthily as possible. The problems with your skin may be a reflection of your body struggling to cope with hormone changes. The skin can be regarded as an organ of detoxification. For example, sweating is an essential process designed to eliminate waste products through your skin. Contained in this fluid, which is secreted by the sweat glands, are salt (sodium chloride) and urea. Sweating is your body's way of getting rid of nitrogenous waste and at the same time controlling your body temperature.

In order to keep the skin healthy you need to eat as 'cleanly' as possible, avoiding fatty foods, and those with additives, artificial sweeteners, colourings and chemicals in general. Make sure that you are drinking enough liquid (at least a litre a day) in the form of water or herbal teas.

With any skin problems it is important to support your liver. The liver is the waste disposal unit of the body, not only for toxins, but also for hormones and other waste products. Follow the recommendations on page 77 for keeping your liver healthy and add in the herbs milk thistle and dandelion. These can be taken together in tincture form (1 teaspoon three times a day throughout your cycle, stopping when you have your period). Take this blend for three months while you 'clean' up your diet and balance your blood sugar.

And last but not least is the mineral zinc, which is one of the most important nutrients for the skin. It is already known that women with PMS can be deficient in zinc[20] and zinc is crucial for general hormone balance. It is especially important in keeping testosterone in balance.

If you suffer from any premenstrual skin problems, add in a total of 30mg of zinc per day for three months. After this period, go back to a multivitamin and mineral tablet alone and assess how well your skin is doing.

While you are waiting for your skin to improve through diet, herbs and supplements, you can also use tea-tree oil to dab on any spots. This oil (*Melaleuca alternifolia*) has excellent antiseptic, anti-bacterial and anti-fungal properties.

Skin problems can also be linked to food allergies, particularly when you may be more sensitive to certain foods premenstrually. For more information on testing for food allergies, see pages 169–70.

There are a number of useful homeopathic remedies for premenstrual skin problems, including:

• Nux vomica, for spots made worse by alcohol, tea and coffee. You may be constipated and irritable.

- Hepar sulph, for large spots that look like boils and are painful to touch
- Pulsatilla, when there is bloating, and you feel tearful.

Tiredness and fatigue

Tiredness is a major problem for many women and can be an underlying problem throughout the entire cycle, becoming much worse before your period. There is now a recognised medical condition called TATT (tired all the time), but all this does put a label on a problem it does not explain why it occurs or what can be done about it.

Some women have told me that they know when their period is due because they feel absolutely exhausted a few days beforehand.

As fatigue is one of the key PMS symptoms, all the factors that are associated with the condition need to be considered. This includes blood sugar fluctuations and hormone changes.

If lack of energy and fatigue are a major problem, run through this checklist.

Are your iron and thyroid (see pages 159–62) levels normal?

It's a good idea to rule out these problems in advance. See your doctor if you are persistently tired and suffer from the symptoms associated with these problems.

Are you sleeping well?

If you not sleeping properly, you will not have enough energy to get through the day. Take on board all of the recommendations for getting a good night's sleep (see pages 88–90).

Are you drinking tea or coffee during the day?

You might think that caffeine will keep you going, but in the long term it will actually make you feel more tired. Eliminate all caffeine from your diet.

Are you eating little and often?

Food is your body's fuel. It is much the same concept as putting petrol in the car. You need to eat regularly to make sure your body has enough fuel, and also to ensure that your blood sugar is balanced. One of the main symptoms of blood sugar fluctuations is fatigue, so follow all the recommendations on pages 48–57.

Are you stressed?

Adrenaline will prevent your hormones from being properly used in the lead-up to your period, making your PMS symptoms, particularly fatigue, that much worse. Follow the suggestions on pages 81–6 for dealing with stress.

Are you getting enough exercise?

This is often a problem, and it's not surprising. You may feel so tired during the premenstrual period that you simply do not have the energy to exercise. However, it can be just what you need to feel invigorated and full of energy again. It can also help with other symptoms of PMS (see pages 92–4). The best option in this situation is to go for a long walk in the fresh air, which gives your brain and body the oxygen it needs to lift the feelings of fatigue.

Could you have candida?

If the fatigue persists, you may need to rule out candida (pages 154–9 and 166) and/or a food allergy (pages 169–70) which may be exacerbated premenstrually.

Natural remedies

Co-enzyme Q10, a substance present in all human tissue and organs, is a vital catalyst in the provision of energy for all our cells. The consequence of a deficiency of co-enzyme Q10 is a reduction in energy. Take 30mg per day of co-enzyme over a period of three months.

The B vitamins are important if you are tired, as one of the deficiency symptoms of the major B vitamins, such as B3, B5 and B6, is lack of energy. See pages 173–4 for details of an appropriate dosage.

Siberian ginseng (*Eleutherococcus senticosus*) is helpful as it works with your own body's needs, providing energy when required, and helping to combat stress and fatigue when you are under pressure. It supports adrenal gland function and acts as a tonic to these glands. Siberian ginseng is extremely useful when you have been under mental or physical stress and should be taken for around three months.

Ginger can revive flagging energy. Use it fresh in food. As a quick pick-me-up, grate ginger into hot water and drink as a tea. Cinnamon could be added, as this spice also helps to raise energy.

Acupuncture combats fatigue effectively by working on the energy channels throughout the body.

Aromatherapy oils such as basil and rosemary can be helpful for mental and physical fatigue. Both are stimulating and rejuvenating. Try them in a vaporiser in your room, or add a few drops in the bath. Any of the oils suggested for stress and sleep will also be helpful (see pages 85–6 and 89).

There are many homeopathic remedies that are indicated for fatigue, and you could try some of the following in the short term:

- Phosphoric acid, when you feel emotionally drained, apathetic and physically exhausted

- Picric acid, which is useful if you feel that you have lost any sense of drive or determination, and lack willpower because you are so tired

- Arsenicum, when you feel restless, chilly, tired and feel that you are constantly fending off anxiety. You may be obsessively neat and tidy, despite fatigue

- China, when you feel chilly, on edge and oversensitive to light, noise and other stimuli. You feel exhausted upon waking

- Nux vomica and Sepia, which are also useful if you feel unusually sleepy in the morning. These are both good 'female' remedies, and deal with many of the symptoms of PMS

Now you have not only the basics of vanquishing PMS, but also a long-term maintenance plan for picking off any negative symptoms that arise during your recovery. What if your condition doesn't improve no matter what you do, though? The next chapter has the answers.

CHAPTER 11

Could There Be Another Cause?

The PMS 'umbrella' covers a huge range of physical symptoms, as we've seen. As you get to grips with treating your symptoms, it's vital to realise that many of these can actually be signs of other health conditions. If the natural treatments for PMS simply do not have the desired effect, it's very likely that there may be something else at the root of the problem.

It's worth looking at some of these other possibilities, if only to rule them out. If any of these symptoms seem familiar, do see your doctor, or follow the natural treatments outlined below.

Candida

If you have tried to get rid of your PMS symptoms and have found that nothing works, it's possible that you're suffering from candida, an overgrowth of yeast. *Candida albicans* is a type of parasitic, yeast-like fungus that inhabits the intestines, genital tract, mouth, oesophagus and throat. Normally this fungus lives in a healthy balance with the other bacteria and yeasts in the body, but certain conditions can cause it to multiply, weakening the immune system and causing an infection known as candidiasis. The fungus can travel throughout the body, via the bloodstream.

In the intestines, the yeast form of candida can become 'mycelial' (that, is, it forms root-like growths). These roots can penetrate the intestine walls, and cause the gut to 'leak'. Small pieces of undigested food then escape into the bloodstream. This condition is known as 'leaky gut syndrome'.

Persistent vaginal thrush can be one of the symptoms of candidiasis, but other symptoms can include food cravings, especially for sugar and bread, fatigue, a bloated stomach with excess flatulence, a 'spaced out' feeling, and becoming tipsy on a very small amount of alcohol. Both men and women can suffer from candidiasis.

Do you suffer from any of these symptoms?

- Sugar cravings
- Cravings for foods such as wine, bread, cheese
- Migraines or headaches
- Chronic thrush
- Inability to lose weight
- Constant tiredness
- Often feeling spaced out
- Feeling drunk on a small amount of alcohol
- Feeling bloated and having flatulence

If these symptoms seem familiar, then you may have candidiasis.

Candida and PMS

One study looked at women with severe PMS who also had a history of vaginal candidiasis, or thrush. All of these women had tried various treatments for PMS, including vitamin B6, drugs and psychotherapy, with no success. They were put on an anti-candida diet and an anti-fungal treatment and found significant relief from their PMS symptoms.[1]

If you suspect that candida is at the root of your problems, you will need to test for candidiasis. Food allergies (see pages 169–70) may need to be checked as well. To do this, you'll need expert advice. Please either contact me (see page 187), or see a nutritional therapist (see page 191) for an individual assessment and treatment plan.

A stool test, which can be organised by post, can be used to detect an overgrowth of yeast in the digestive system. The test also show shows the levels of beneficial bacteria in your body. But don't assume that because you have these symptoms, there is candida present. Many of my patients have believed they were suffering from candidiasis – even going to the extent of following an anti-candida diet for some time – before a stool test showed that a parasitic infestation rather than candida was at the root of their problem. The symptoms of both conditions are remarkably similar, so it is essential that you have the appropriate tests to get the correct treatment.

Your body is teeming with literally millions of bacteria, and under ideal circumstances they are kept in a healthy balance. In other words, the healthy bacteria keep the unhealthy bacteria in check. When your immune system is compromised, say because of illness or a poor diet, the proportion of the different bacteria can alter, allowing yeast (candida) to grow out of control.

When antibiotics are given for infection, they do not discriminate between the 'good' bacteria and the 'bad' bacteria in the body. They wipe out everything, which means that there are not enough of the good bacteria to keep yeast (and other invaders) at bay. What's the result? Candida is no longer controlled and it begins to overgrow.

Taking the Pill alters the levels of natural hormones in the body (including those in the vagina), so you can become more susceptible to thrush. Hormonal changes during pregnancy and before a period can also make you more susceptible to a yeast overgrowth because the environment in the vagina changes.

Note: If you have persistent yeast infections, it's worth checking to see that you are not suffering from diabetes. Regular yeast infections can be an indication of undiagnosed diabetes.

Dietary changes and supplements

You can help to eliminate candida by focusing on a few dietary changes. You will definitely need to avoid sugar and any foods containing sugar, as they will promote the growth of yeast. You also need to cut out foods that contain yeast, and any products that are fermented, such as bread and wine.

Yoghurt Live yoghurt containing the culture acidophilus or bifidus, both of which are found naturally in your gut, is the most beneficial type (see page 70). These cultures represent some of the 'healthy' bacteria, which can help to prevent an overgrowth of yeast in the body. Fruit yoghurts should be avoided because very high sugar content will 'feed' the yeast.

When researchers gave women one *Lactobacillus acidophilus*-containing yoghurt a day over six months, there was a threefold decrease in bouts of thrush.[2]

Along with your general multivitamin and mineral supplement and the other supplements recommended for PMS, it is worth adding in some extra nutrients that are known scientifically to help with candida and boost the immune system. Then your body will be better able to deal with any invaders.

Beta-carotene Levels of beta-carotene (a type of vitamin A) have been found to be low in the vaginal cells of women who have thrush. It is suggested that this may affect the immune response of the cells in the vagina, which encourages (or at least allows) the yeast to overgrow.[3]

Zinc Zinc deficiency has been connected with women who have recurrent thrush.[4] Adequate levels of zinc are critical for the optimum functioning of your immune system. People who are deficient in zinc will be susceptible to recurrent infections or infestations of any kind (that's why you may seem to suffer from one cold or tummy bug after another when you are run down). Your immune system can become compromised and your body will not be able to control yeast overgrowth.

Essential fatty acids (EFAs) The essential fatty acids that are contained in oily fish and in nuts and seeds have anti-fungal, anti-bacterial and anti-viral actions.[5] So it is important to take EFAs in supplements while you are combating candida. If you have a tendency to recurrent thrush, it's worth taking a capsule of linseed oil every day over a period of six months. Try also to ensure that you are getting enough of these essential fats in your food (see pages 59–61).

Garlic Garlic is well known for its effect on the immune system and it has both anti-bacterial and anti-fungal properties. Take garlic as a supplement when you are trying to eliminate candida, and as prevention if you are prone to attacks of thrush. In clinical studies, garlic extracts have been to found to prevent the growth of candida.[6]

One of the active ingredients in garlic is called allicin, and it appears that this is the ingredient that prevents overgrowth of yeast. When buying supplements, choose one with a high level of allicin. Better still, chew a clove of fresh garlic every day, if you can (and if your friends can bear it!). When heated, garlic loses its anti-fungal qualities, so it's worth trying to incorporate raw garlic into your diet in some form, even if it's in salads or salad dressings.

Probiotics A probiotic is the opposite of an antibiotic, which means that it encourages rather than destroys bacteria in the body. That's not as alarming as it sounds! What probiotics do is increase the growth of 'healthy' bacteria in the body, which are known as flora. These in turn help to control the amount of yeast overgrowth. As well as eating live plain organic yoghurt, it is important to take supplements of *Lactobacillus acidophilus,* one of the best-known and most effective probiotics. Yoghurt has been shown to be helpful in *preventing* attacks of candida, but a probiotic supplement goes one step further to actually *treat* a candida infection. The difference is that lactobacillus levels in yoghurt are high enough to work on a preventative basis, but they will not be concentrated enough to deal with an infection. Make sure the one you buy has to be kept in the refrigerator, because these are viable cells that need to be kept at a low temperature.

Some companies make a vaginal cream containing the beneficial bacteria, which can be inserted directly into the vagina with an applicator. This is appropriate for vaginal candida. There are also acidophilus capsules that can be inserted into the vagina. Alternatively, you can use live yoghurt in the same way. Some women slather a tampon with yoghurt, and insert it into their vaginas, removing the tampon after thirty minutes or so, which should be enough time for the yoghurt with all its beneficial bacteria to be absorbed by the body. This method can be effective but, like anything that is used internally, messy! Furthermore, if you already have a yeast infection, there can be no doubt that your levels of beneficial bacteria are not high enough. Even if you choose one of these methods, it's a good idea to take a good probiotic alongside.

If you are currently suffering from thrush, add in fructo-oligosaccharides (FOS), which are the naturally occurring water-soluble fibre in fruits and vegetables. These act as a food source for the growth of friendly bacteria.

Herbs

In this context, the herbs we'll look at treat an active attack of thrush and also work to prevent future attacks of candida.

Goldenseal (*Hydrastis canadensis*) This is the herb of choice for vaginal thrush, and, indeed, candida in general, because it contains a substance called berberine, which acts both to stimulate the immune system and to combat yeasts and bacteria.[7] It has become an endangered herb because of overuse, so if you can't obtain it then use barberry root bark (*Berberis vulgaris*) instead.

Calendula (*Calendula officinalis*) This herb is also known as pot marigold, and works as an anti-fungal agent, which is very beneficial when treating yeast. It is also anti-microbial, so can be helpful when fighting any kind of infection.

Pau d'arco (*Tabebuia impetiginosa*) This is a brilliant herb for candida because it has both immune-enhancing and anti-fungal properties. In order for it to be effective you need a product from the whole bark of the tree *Tabebuia impetiginosa*. Some products contain only the active ingredient, lapachol. If this is taken in high doses, it can cause nausea and vomiting. This is another example (see page 110), of the need to use the plant as nature supplies it: using the active ingredient alone can result in side-effects. When you take pau d'arco as a tincture made from the whole bark, there are no side-effects.

Tea-tree oil (*Melaleuca alternifolia*) Research has been undertaken into the effects of tea-tree oil on candida and other vaginal infections.[8] The herb has been shown to be an excellent anti-fungal and anti-bacterial agent.

This essential oil (the same type of oil that is used in aromatherapy) is not taken by mouth, but used vaginally to combat thrush. It is possible to buy tea-tree oil pessaries from a healthfood shop. Try adding a few drops of tea-tree essential oil to your bath when you have thrush. If you are prone to thrush or any manifestation of candida, it can be used on a preventative basis.

Echinacea Because your immunity will be compromised if you suffer from candida, one of the aims of herbal treatment will be to boost your immune system.

Echinacea is one of the best herbs for toning up the immune system. One study showed that women suffering from recurrent thrush who were given echinacea had a 43 per cent reduction in the number of attacks.[9]

For optimum benefit to the immune system, it seems that echinacea is more effective if you take short regular breaks from it. I would suggest ten days on and three days off.

Thyroid function

The thyroid gland situated in your neck helps control your metabolism. It produces two hormones, thyroxine and triidothyronine. These hormones are released when a message is sent from the hypothalamus and the pituitary gland, which also produces thyroid-stimulating hormones (TSH) and thyrotrophin-releasing hormones.

The thyroid gland is like a thermostat that regulates your body temperature by secreting these two hormones, which control how quickly the body burns calories and uses energy. An underactive thyroid, a condition known as hypothyroidism, is a deficiency of thyroid hormone caused by one of two things: either your pituitary gland is not producing TSH, or your thyroid is not working properly.

It has been found that a large percentage of women with PMS have low thyroid function (hypothyroidism).[10] This can be so striking that in one study, 51 out of 54 women with PMS had low thyroid function, whereas none of the 12 women in the study without PMS had low thyroid function. But again, as with anything to do with PMS, you can find the opposite: other research has only shown it to be slightly more common.[11]

PMS symptoms can be similar to those of thyroid problems so thyroid diagnosis can be missed. It is important that your thyroid is checked; it has been found that if women have both symptoms of PMS and low thyroid function, treating the thyroid problem will alleviate the PMS symptoms altogether.[12]

Pinning down a thyroid problem

If you answer 'yes' to four or more of the following questions, your thyroid gland could be underactive. Visit your doctor for a blood test, which can establish how well your thyroid is functioning.

- Has your weight gone up gradually over months for no apparent reason?
- Do you often feel cold?
- Are you constipated?
- Are you depressed, forgetful or confused?
- Are you losing hair or is it drier than it used to be?
- Are you having menstrual problems?
- Are you having difficulty getting pregnant?
- Have you noticed a lack of energy?
- Are you getting headaches?

If a blood test does not show that you have an underactive thyroid, you may only have a mild problem, which could go undetected in a blood test. The other way to test whether you have low thyroid function is to measure your temperature. If it is too low, it may indicate that you have a sluggish metabolism caused by an underactive thyroid.

Take your temperature once a day for three days. If you are having periods, take your temperature on the second, third and fourth days of the cycle. A woman's body temperature rises after ovulation, so it would not give a clear picture if done later in the cycle. If you are not menstruating, take your temperature on any three consecutive days.

Put a thermometer by your bed before you go to sleep; a mercury thermometer is fine but there are some good electronic ones on the market. When you wake, lie still in bed and take your temperature before drinking or visiting the bathroom. Put the thermometer in your armpit and leave it until it bleeps. If you are using a mercury thermometer, leave it for ten minutes.

If your average temperature over the three days falls below 36.4°C (97.6°F), your thyroid may be under-functioning.

Conventional treatments

If a blood test shows that your thyroid is not functioning properly, you would normally be given thyroxine. Side-effects are usually only a problem if it is given in excessively high doses, and it is normal procedure for you to be monitored to check you are taking the correct dose.

The difficulty is that many times an underactive thyroid problem may not be accurately diagnosed because your doctor may simply not test for it. It may also not be diagnosed because the blood tests look normal – even though you're feeling all the symptoms. This can happen when the thyroid gland is producing enough hormones, but the cells that are supposed to latch on to the hormones are not picking them up. That's just one reason why the temperature test can be so useful.

Natural treatments

Diet Some foods, called goitrogens, can block the uptake of iodine and so worsen an underactive thyroid problem. These include turnips, cabbage, peanuts, soya, pine nuts and millet. These foods only seem to be a problem when they are eaten raw and in large amounts, so make sure they are cooked well and eat in moderation.

On the other hand, foods such as seaweeds, which are low in calories, have a very high mineral content, including the trace minerals zinc, manganese, chromium, selenium and cobalt, and the macro minerals calcium, magnesium, iron and iodine. Iodine is of particular importance, as it is essential for the healthy functioning of the thyroid gland. Scientific studies have shown that the consumption of seaweed can also have anti-cancer benefits[13] and can reduce cholesterol and improve fat metabolism.[14] (I also discuss seaweed under 'Herbs', below.)

If you would like to know how to cook using seaweed, see my book *Natural Alternatives to HRT Cookbook*.

Selenium This is a very useful mineral for treating an underactive thyroid, as it helps thyroid hormones function properly. Low levels of selenium have been linked to underactive thyroid problems.[15] Take 100 mcg per day.

Other nutrients It is important that you take a good multivitamin and mineral supplement because a number of other nutrients play a vital part in healthy thyroid function. These include zinc, vitamin A, vitamin E, the B vitamins (especially B3 and B6), vitamin C and also essential fatty acids such as linseed and fish oil.

Herbs The two hormones produced by the thyroid gland, thyroxine and triidothyronine, are made from iodine and the amino acid tyrosine. Naturally rich sources of iodine are seafoods, especially saltwater fish, and seaweeds such as kelp. Herbalists have traditionally used the seaweed bladderwrack (*Fucus vesiculosus*) to help with an underactive thyroid. It is normally taken as a tablet, but if you are lucky enough to be able to buy it fresh or dried, you can make an infusion by pouring a cup of boiling water onto 10 to 15ml (2 to 3 teaspoons) of dried bladderwrack and leaving it for 10 minutes. This infusion can be drunk three times a day.

> **Warning:** if you take too much iodine, then this can actually make an underactive thyroid worse. It is recommended that you see a qualified practitioner for help with thyroid problems.

Diabetes and blood sugar problems

We've seen how vital it is to balance blood sugar in treating PMS. One blood sugar disorder is hypoglycaemia, a condition that occurs when there is a low level of glucose (sugar) in the blood. We discussed the various causes of low blood sugar on page 49.

Left unchecked, blood sugar problems – including hypoglycaemia – can lead to diabetes, and many of the symptoms of diabetes mimic those of

PMS. This may seem confusing. Diabetes is obviously a problem associated with high blood sugar levels, which is the opposite of hypoglycaemia. But there are two different kinds of diabetes: Type I (also called insulin dependent diabetes or juvenile diabetes) and Type II (also called non-insulin dependent or late-onset [middle age] diabetes). Hypoglycaemia, as we'll see in a bit, is a key player in the second kind.

Type I diabetes usually occurs early in life, as the result of an inability of the pancreas to produce insulin. Daily injections of insulin have to be given to prevent serious health problems and even death.

The insulin controls the amount of glucose in the bloodstream. The amount of insulin needed by an individual is carefully monitored. Otherwise they will swing from periods of very high blood glucose levels (hyperglycaemia, where either not enough insulin is used or a meal produced excessively high glucose levels) to very low blood glucose levels (hypoglycaemia, where too much insulin has been injected or a meal has been skipped after insulin was used).

Type II diabetes is much more widespread than Type I, counting for up to 90 per cent of all cases of diabetes and steadily increasing, even in young people. This scenario was, literally, unheard of just a few years ago. In this case, the problem is not that the pancreas doesn't produce enough insulin – in fact, it often provides high levels of insulin. The issue here is the fact that the body does not respond to it. This condition is known as 'insulin resistance'. That is, insulin levels are high (hyperinsulinaemia), but the insulin cannot transport glucose into the cells. This, in turn, leads to high levels of blood glucose (sugar). So the pancreas pumps out more insulin to get glucose into the cells. Over time, however, the pancreas may not be able to keep up this output, in which case it may eventually be unable to produce enough insulin to sustain normal levels.

Here's how hypoglycaemia enters the picture. The type of hypoglycaemia that we have discussed in this book is triggered by eating foods that enter the bloodstream very quickly, causing a fast rise in blood sugar. The pancreas then increases its secretion of insulin to match this rise in blood sugar, causing blood sugar to drop rapidly. Adrenaline is then released by the adrenal glands to increase the blood sugar, causing the symptoms listed on page 47. Over time, this places enormous pressure on the adrenal glands, which become exhausted. The same problem affects the pancreas. When the pancreas is exhausted, it cannot produce adequate insulin or it produces too much. In either case, the body cannot respond because it has become resistant to its own insulin. This is Type II diabetes, and it's on the increase.

When you suffer from Type II diabetes, your body is effectively saying 'I can't cope with these roller-coaster rides of blood sugar any more.' This is one reason why it is also called 'adult-onset' diabetes, because it normally occurs after the age of about forty, when the body has had many years of swinging blood sugar levels. When we are younger our bodies can cope with the demands we place upon them, but as we age, it can no longer 'spring back', and all of its systems are affected.

Type II diabetes responds well to dietary intervention, but drugs may need to be used to help the body to become sensitive to insulin again, so that it can use what is actually being produced. Or insulin may be used when the pancreas has been so overworked it can't produce enough.

In any case, if you are experiencing symptoms such as frequent urination, excessive thirst or increased appetite, it is important that you see your doctor to rule out diabetes. If you are given the all-clear, it is crucial that you follow the recommendations in this book not only to eliminate your premenstrual symptoms but to help to prevent any problems in the future, especially if there is a history of Type II diabetes in your family.

CHAPTER 12

Tests

Through the chapters of this book I've outlined problems associated with nutritional deficiencies and health conditions that may be causing or exacerbating your PMS symptoms. You may be wondering how to discover whether any of these problems actually affect you.

Twenty-first-century life proceeds at sprint pace, and most of us have little time to consider our diets carefully. Even when we do eat well, our food is likely to be deficient in the vitamins and minerals we need to keep our bodies healthy and well-balanced. But there's more. Health also depends on how well we are able to absorb and digest the nutrients we eat.

Vitamins and minerals work in balance with one another. For this reason, it is vital that you take the right ones in the right amounts, and in the right combinations at the right times. You will notice that I've recommended a multivitamin and mineral as part of your PMS supplement programme. This provides a good, solid foundation containing all of the key nutrients. All nutrients work in harmony, and if you take one on its own, such as zinc, you can affect the whole overall balance in your body.

But you may also have a minor or major nutritional deficiency at the root of your problems which will require extra supplementation. Below you'll find tests that will find out just what those deficiencies may be. There are also tests to assess whether or not you have a hormone imbalance, a food allergy or candida, or even whether your stress levels are too high. These tests can be crucial in diagnosing a problem that underpins your susceptibility to PMS and all its symptoms.

For information on any of these tests, please contact me through 'Staying in Touch', page 187.

Testing for an imbalance in female hormones

This is a very simple test done on saliva that looks at the pattern of your main female hormones over one cycle and investigates whether there is an imbalance, especially in the second half of the cycle. The test is performed at home and then sent to a lab for analysis. A total of eleven saliva samples are collected over one cycle at specific times.

This test can be done even if you have irregular cycles, and is very useful if there is a suspicion that you have a hormonal imbalance between oestrogen and progesterone, which may be causing the premenstrual symptoms.

Testing for candida

This is an important test, as it has been shown that women with severe PMS who also have a history of vaginal candidiasis or thrush experience relief when put on an anti-candida diet, and given an anti-fungal treatment.[1]

It is possible to test for yeast (candida) overgrowth. You can have yeast overgrowth in the vagina, which is more commonly known as thrush, but it is also possible to have it in other parts of the body. Candida can form in the intestines, for instance (see page 154).

Persistent vaginal thrush can be one of the symptoms of candidiasis, but other symptoms can include food cravings, especially for sugar and bread, fatigue, a bloated stomach with excess flatulence, a 'spaced out' feeling, and becoming tipsy on a very small amount of alcohol. Both men and women can suffer from candidiasis.

A stool test, which can be organised by post, can be used to detect an overgrowth of yeast in the digestive system. This test will look for any kind of yeast – not only candida – because there are many different forms of yeast infection. The test also shows the levels of beneficial bacteria in your body (in other words, the probiotics, such as acidophilus). This stool test also checks for parasitic infestation, as the symptoms can be similar to a candida overgrowth.

Stress index

This is an important test in connection with PMS because of the link between the adrenal glands and your body's ability to use progesterone effectively (see page 48). The test looks at your stress levels by measuring the secretion of hormones from the adrenal glands. The adrenal glands do not secrete their hormones at a constant level during the day. The highest amount is released in the morning and the lowest at night.

The reproductive system is particularly susceptible to stress, and in the extreme, your periods may cease or become irregular. Your immune system and your thyroid function can also be compromised if the adrenal glands are not doing their job properly.

This test measures the rhythm of the adrenal glands by using four saliva samples over a day, which are collected at home and then sent to a lab for analysis.

Mineral analysis

Have you ever gone into a healthfood shop and looked at the array of supplements on the shelves and wondered what you should be taking? There are, in fact, scientific laboratory tests that can evaluate your nutritional status.

There are many ways of testing nutrient deficiencies – for example, by using a sample of blood or sweat. But one of the most cost-effective and convenient ways is through a hair sample. Hair has been shown to reflect a good long-term record of our mineral and nutritional experience.[2] In fact, it's possible that hair samples will eventually be used to screen for potential diabetes or breast cancer. Work is being undertaken in Australia by Professor Veronica James at the University of New South Wales.[3] She analyses hair with a technique called X-ray diffraction. As X-rays are fired through the hair they form a pattern on photographic film. From this pattern the researchers are able to pick up different information. For instance, sugar binds onto the hair filaments of a diabetic patient. It will therefore look different from a strand of hair from a person without diabetes.

Hair samples can also be used to test for drug use, such as cocaine, amphetamines and cannabis. This is helpful in forensic medicine and pathology, to determine whether someone was under the influence of drugs in an accident.

Because your hair cells are some of the fastest-growing cells in the body, they can 'lock' in information about your exposure to certain nutrients as they grow. In this way, your hair forms a permanent record of exposure to beneficial and toxic elements. Analysing hair is an excellent way to test for heavy toxic metals and is used in many medical studies to assess exposure to metals like mercury.[4]

Other ways of testing (using blood or urine, for example) can be less reliable, because the results are influenced by what you may have eaten. Also, your body tries to keep everything in balance. To do this, it tops up the levels of nutrients in your blood by taking them from elsewhere. For instance, if your blood calcium levels fall, your body will pinch calcium from your bones to keep the level constant. A blood test may then suggest that your calcium levels are fine. But a hair analysis showing high levels of calcium would help identify the leaching of calcium from your bones.

However, like any testing medium, hair analysis has its limitations. For instance, when testing for nutrients, it is important that your hair is not contaminated by tints, highlights or perms. Certain minerals (iron, for instance) are best tested using a blood sample. But levels of trace elements can be higher in hair, which make them easier to analyse. Also, because hair doesn't need specialised sampling equipment or storage, this form of testing is accessible for women who are not conveniently near a qualified practitioner.

Hair can be used to analyse levels of calcium, magnesium, zinc, selenium, copper, manganese, chromium and also the toxic metals mercury, aluminium and cadmium.

Once the person's mineral levels have been analysed they are usually asked to fill out a detailed questionnaire. Then a personalised programme of supplements can be offered. It is recommended that this programme is followed for a minimum of three to four months and then the hair is re-tested. Once the mineral and toxic levels are back to normal, it's recommended that you follow a maintenance programme and continue to eat well.

What can the mineral analysis show?

This analysis can show straightforward deficiencies of minerals such as low levels of zinc or selenium. Levels of some minerals (such as copper) can be high, perhaps owing to previous use of the Pill, IUD (coil), or fertility drugs. High levels of copper are a concern, as these are often associated with low zinc levels. Zinc is an important mineral in terms of the reproductive system. Keen swimmers should, however, beware! Swimming can confuse the analysis, showing unusually high levels of copper because the pools are treated with algicides which alter the copper levels.

The results of the mineral tests are given to you as a graph so you can see how far your levels differ from the norm.

Apart from detecting imbalances in the minerals, the tests may show that the toxic metal levels may be too high. If so, two things will be needed. First of all, you will need to try to work out the source of contamination – and avoid it if possible. Secondly, you'll need to take specific nutrients, such as antioxidants, to eliminate the toxins from your body.

Nutritional questionnaire

This questionnaire is usually done in conjunction with the mineral analysis. You are asked about your daily eating habits, your lifestyle, symptoms, health problems and risk factors. Each vitamin and mineral has certain deficiency symptoms, so a lack of vitamin C, for example, can give you frequent infections, easy bruising, bleeding gums and slow wound healing. When you complete this comprehensive questionnaire you will be sent a detailed report showing which of the twelve vitamins (A, D, E, C, B1, B2, B3, B5, B6, B12, folic acid and biotin), seven minerals (calcium, magnesium, zinc, manganese, chromium, copper and selenium) and essential fatty acids you need to take. This report will tell you what quantities you need in order to bring your body back into balance and optimum health.

Allergy/food intolerance test

If you suffer from migraines or headaches this is a useful test, as it is used to track down a food trigger (see pages 137–8). There are two types of allergic reactions. Type A (classic allergy) is diagnosed when your reaction takes place immediately after contact with an allergen, such as peanuts. Type B (delayed allergy or intolerance) is diagnosed when the reaction takes place between one hour and four days after contact with the allergen. Common Type B allergens include dairy produce, eggs, wheat and sugar. Symptoms such as weight gain, bloating, water retention, fatigue, aching joints and headaches can all be due to a Type B allergy.

It is now possible to have a blood test that analyses 217 different foods and food additives by measuring the release of certain chemicals that are responsible for the symptoms of food intolerance. You would then know the foods to which you are reacting, and these can be avoided for a short period of time. Unlike with a Type A allergy, these foods would not have to avoided indefinitely. While you are avoiding the foods, the aim would be to strengthen and correct any digestive problems so that afterwards you can eat in moderation the foods to which you are intolerant.

When food is not being digested properly (see below), food particles can leak out into the bloodstream. Instead of seeing these particles as food, your body views them as toxins and sets up an immune system reaction to them. This is often caused by sheer overload – in other words, eating too much of the same foods too often. Wheat is often the culprit because you can end up eating it throughout the day – for example, toast for breakfast, a sandwich for lunch, pasta in the evening, and biscuits in between.

The test is analysed from a sample of blood and a kit can be sent to enable your practice nurse or doctor to take a small quantity of blood. This is sent to the laboratory and, after it has been analysed, you are sent an extensive personalised report outlining:

- Foods that are highly reactive for you, those that are borderline and those that are OK
- Recommendations of how to implement food changes and how to reintroduce the reactive/borderline foods safely at a later date.

Testing for a leaky gut

Tracking down the foods to which you may be sensitive is only solving half the problem. Why has the problem developed in the first place? What happens when you re-introduce the offending foods? The answer lies in the state of your gut, and its capacity to process food properly. And allergies and food intolerances are often a symptom that all is not well with your digestive system.

If your intestines are not functioning properly, you may not be absorbing nutrients efficiently, which means you can become deficient in vital vitamins and minerals. By checking your urine a lab can assess the state of your digestive system.

All food must be broken down by the digestive system, then pass into the bloodstream and be dealt with by the body's lymphatic system. If this doesn't happen in the right way, the body 'sees' normal food as an antigen, a toxin, and sets up an immune system reaction to deal with it. At the same time, this undigested food is sitting around fermenting and putrefying.

Large spaces can develop between the cells in the gut wall and food molecules can then pass into the bloodstream. This is called leaky gut or intestinal permeability and can result in the overgrowth of candida (see page 154).

Initially it is important to stop eating the offending foods, which will help to alleviate the symptoms and make you feel better. Then the whole environment of the gut needs to be healed as well, in order to get the intestinal bacteria back in balance again so that you can stay healthy and prevent the symptoms from recurring.

This condition has only recently become widely recognised, and this very effective non-invasive urine test is relatively new. It can be done in your own home with a kit that is posted to you. Two urine samples are required. The first one is a pre-test sample and the second is taken six hours after drinking a special liquid which contains two marker molecules. When the samples are analysed, the amount of the marker molecules detected by the laboratory will give a strong indication of how permeable – that is, leaky – your gut is. Once you have this information, you can decide what the best course of action will be in order to heal your intestines.

CHAPTER 13

Putting It All Together

In this section you'll get help on the right way to start eliminating your premenstrual symptoms.

What do you do if you are already taking medication for PMS?

If you would like to try the natural approach, you will need to speak to your doctor about stopping your medication. This is important because some drugs, such as antidepressants, should not be discontinued suddenly. If you have to wait for a few months before coming off the medication, take on board all of the dietary recommendations and remember to take the vitamins and minerals recommended. Do not begin the herb programme until you have stopped taking your drugs.

If your PMS is worse on the Pill, or started when you began taking the Pill, think seriously about using another form of contraception. You can still put the dietary advice in place and take the vitamins and minerals recommended below, but you may just be fighting a losing battle. Your PMS may actually be *caused* by the hormones you are putting into your body. Don't take any of the herbs suggested when you are on the Pill, unless you are under the supervision of a registered, experienced practitioner.

The natural approach to PMS is very successful, so I would recommend that you try it over a period of three months. You do not have anything to lose except your symptoms. Change your diet, add in the supplements and take the herbs. At the end of the three months, still keep eating sensibly most of the time; obviously you don't need to be so strict but you also don't want the symptoms to return. You could stop the herbs at the end of the three months and also the supplements, except for the multivitamin and mineral.

Your diet

Remember, balancing your blood sugar is one of the most important elements of the PMS diet (see pages 48–57). Therefore, eliminate anything that causes rapid changes in blood sugar – such as coffee, tea, sugar, alcohol and chocolate – and make sure that you are eating little and often. The second aim of the PMS diet is to restore your body to a healthy balance by ensuring that it gets the tools it needs to work at optimum level. When you eat healthily, you are providing the foundation of good health. Everything we eat is used to create bones, tissue and muscles, and to help our bodies to function. It goes without saying that a junk-food diet will provide suboptimal nutrition for these purposes.

Your supplement plan

The following supplement programme should be taken over the next three months, while you are also changing your eating habits. This will help to correct any deficiencies and give you those nutrients that are particularly important for the elimination of PMS symptoms.

- A good multivitamin and mineral supplement
- Vitamin B6 (as pyridoxal-5-phosphate, at 50mg per day)
- Vitamin E (as d-alpha tocopherol, at 300iu per day)
- Magnesium citrate or amino acid chelate (200mg per day)
- Zinc citrate (15mg per day)
- GLA (150mg per day)

As mentioned on page 108, the multivitamin and mineral supplement is necessary to give you 'a bit of everything'. In the case of PMS, it also gives you all the B vitamins, calcium and manganese you need to help overcome the problem. Instead of purchasing a number of different supplements, all of which have their role in the body, you will get the majority of what you need from a single multivitamin and mineral supplement.

Vitamin B6, vitamin E, magnesium, zinc and GLA have been added in on top of the multivitamin and mineral supplement because they are needed at higher levels than would be contained in the multi alone.

Note: Each nutrient represents the total intake for one day, so if your multivitamin and mineral contains 25mg of vitamin B6, you only need to add 25mg in a separate supplement form.

Herbs

Herbs are helpful over the first three months to correct any hormone imbalances.

Use a tincture of equal parts agnus–castus, black cohosh, and skullcap. Take 1 teaspoon three times a day and stop when you have your period.

To make this programme simpler, I have formulated a product called PM Comfort made by The Natural Health Practice, which contains all the nutrients and herbs mentioned above. It is designed so that you do not need to hunt around all the different brands to find the correct levels of nutrients: it has been specifically formulated to contain everything you need in one pack. There are three vegetarian capsules. One is a multivitamin and mineral containing excellent amounts of all the vitamins and minerals you need to give you a good foundation, including vitamin E and zinc. The second capsule gives extra magnesium and B6 and also contains the correct amount of GLA, as recommended above. The third capsule contains the most beneficial herbs for PMS, including milk thistle (see pages 114–15) to give your liver support over the first three months. All the nutrients are of the highest quality in their most absorbable form to ensure you get the maximum benefit from them. If you can't get this locally then call 01892 750511 or email health@marilynglenville.com and it can be posted to you.

Extras

I have listed below some extra useful herbs and supplements that may be necessary if you have very strong, specific premenstrual symptoms. I would suggest that you add these to the basic programme.

For food or sugar cravings

• Chromium at 200mcg per day (including the chromium in your multi)

- *Garcinia cambogia*, which contains HCA (hydroxy-citric acid – see page 133). There should be approximately 250mg of HCA in each capsule. Take just before lunch and dinner.

Some companies make a combination supplement of chromium and HCA, which is useful.

Note: Do not take the HCA if you have a problem with migraines. Only add chromium to your supplement programme.

For water retention

Use dandelion, taking 1 teaspoon three times a day and stopping when you have your period.

For migraines or headaches

The herb milk thistle which is an excellent herb for the liver can be extremely helpful for migraines and headaches. Take 1 teaspoon three times a day and stop when you have your period.

For depression

- This is a very common premenstrual symptom. While you are changing your diet, add 50g of 5-HTP (5-hydroxytryptophan – see page 91). Take three times per day with meals.
- St John's wort – 1 teaspoon three times a day, stopping when you bleed.

For stress

Because of the connection with the adrenal glands and PMS, you may often be stressed, so add in:

- Siberian ginseng, taking 1 teaspoon three times a day. Stop when you have your period.

For other symptoms

Throughout the book we have focused on some of the most common symptoms related to PMS, and suggested nutrients and supplements that will ease them. If for some reason your symptoms are not completely eased by the programme I have suggested, please contact me for details of a nutritional therapist, have a postal consultation or come and see me, to assess whether there are other problems at the root of your PMS. You may also wish to consult a homeopath, who will be able to prescribe remedies according to your individual constitution.

Important Points to Remember

- Always investigate the cause of symptoms before taking any drugs, or beginning a natural treatment programme.
- Keep a diary of symptoms, making a note of when they occur. If they always occur in the weeks before your period, but stop when your period begins, they are undoubtedly associated with PMS.
- Follow the dietary recommendations.
- Avoid caffeine, especially if you suffer from breast problems.
- Stop taking the Pill if your symptoms came on when you began taking it. Choose another form of contraception instead.
- Take steps to balance your blood sugar levels. This means giving up refined carbohydrate products in favour of wholegrain, wholemeal complex carbohydrates. Eat little and often.
- Have a complex-carbohydrate-rich, protein-poor evening meal.
- Include a good source of essential fatty acids (see page 59–61) in your diet.
- Take supplements for three months.
- Take herbs that help balance your hormones for three months.
- Take any extra supplements or herbs on top of the basic programme if you have more specific symptoms.
- Begin a regular exercise programme, which has a positive effect on PMS symptoms.
- Take care of your liver!
- Take steps to deal with any stress in your life.

Notes

Part One: The PMS Puzzle

Introduction

1 Magos, A.L. et al. 'Treatment of the pre-menstrual syndrome by subcutaneous oestradiol implants and cyclical oral noresthisterone: placebo controlled study.' *British Medical Journal, Clinical Research Edition*, vol 292, no 6536, pp. 1629–33 (1986).

2 'American College of Obstetrics and Gynaecology Opinion: Pre-menstrual syndrome.' *International Journal of Gynaecology and Obstetrics*, vol 50, pp. 80–4 (1995).

3 Schagen van Leeuwen, J.H. et al. 'Is pre-menstrual syndrome an endocrine disorder?' *Journal of Psychosomatic Obstetrics and Gynaecology*, vol 14, no 2, pp. 91–109 (1993).

Chapter 1: What Is PMS?

1 Clare, A. 'Pre-menstrual syndrome: Single or multiple causes?' *Canadian Journal of Psychiatry*, vol 30, pp. 474–82 (1985).

2 Maudsley, H. *Body and Mind*. Macmillan, London (1873).

3 Clare. 'Pre-menstrual syndrome.'

4 Clare. 'Pre-menstrual syndrome.'

5 Greene, R. and Dalton, K. 'The pre-menstrual syndrome.' *British Medical Journal*, BMJ 1 (1953).

6 'American College of Obstetrics and Gynaecology Opinion: Pre-menstrual syndrome.' *International Journal of Gynaecology and Obstetrics*, vol 50, pp. 80–4 (1995).

7 Abraham, G.E. 'Nutritional factors in the aetiology of the pre-menstrual tension syndromes.' *Journal of Reproductive Medicine*, vol 28, no 7, pp. 446–64 (1983).

8 Schmidt, P.J. et al. 'Differential behavioural effects of gonadal steroids in women with and in those without pre-menstrual syndrome.' *New England Journal of Medicine*, vol 338, no 4, pp. 209–16 (1998).

9 Dalton, K. *Pre-menstrual Syndrome Goes to Court*. Peter Andrew Publishing Co., Worcestershire (1990).

10 Dalton, K. 'Menstruation and acute psychiatric illness.' *British Medical Journal*, vol 1, pp. 148–9 (1959).

11 Dalton, K. 'Menstruation and accidents.' *British Medical Journal*, vol 2, 1425–6 (1960).

12 Dalton, K. 'Children's hospital admissions and mother's menstruation.' *British Medical Journal*, vol 2, pp. 27–8 (1970).

Chapter 2: The Cause of PMS

1 Halbreich, U. 'Menstrually related disorder: what we do know, what we only believe that we know and what we know that we do not know.' *Critical Reviews in Neurobiology*, vol 9, pp. 163–75 (1995).

2 Facchinetti, F. et al. 'Oestradiol/progesterone imbalance and the pre-menstrual syndrome.' *Lancet*, vol 2, p. 1302 (1983).

3 Abraham, G.E. 'Pre-menstrual tension.' *Problems in Obstetrics and Gynaecology*, vol 3, no 12, pp. 1–39 (1980).

4 Smith, R.N. et al. 'A randomised comparison over 8 months of 100mcg and 200mcg twice weekly doses of transdermal oestradiol in the treatment of severe pre-menstrual syndrome.' *British Journal of Obstetrics and Gynaecology*, vol 102, pp. 475–84 (1995).

5 Abraham, G.E. 'Nutritional factors in the aetiology of the pre-menstrual tension syndromes.' *Journal of Reproductive Medicine*, vol 28, pp. 446–64 (1983).

6 Clare, A. 'Pre-menstrual syndrome: single or multiple causes?' *Canadian Journal of Psychiatry*, vol 30, pp. 474–82 (1985).

7 Abraham, G.E. 'Role of nutrition in managing the pre-menstrual tension syndromes.' *Journal of Reproductive Medicine*, vol 32, no 6, pp. 405–22 (1987).

8 Brayshaw, N.D. and Brayshaw, D.D. 'Thyroid hypofunction in pre-menstrual syndrome.' *New England Journal of Medicine*, vol 315, pp. 1486–7 (1986).

9 Schmidt et al. 'Thyroid function in women with pre-menstrual syndrome.' *The Journal of Clinical Endocrinology and Metabolism*, vol 76, pp. 671–4 (1993).

10 Eriksson, E. et al. 'Serum levels of androgens are higher in women with pre-menstrual irritability and dysphoria than in controls.' *Psychoneuroimmunology*, vol 17, no 2–3, pp. 195–204 (1992).

11 Clare. 'Pre-menstrual syndrome.'

12 Stewart, A. 'Clinical and biochemical effects of nutritional supplementation on the pre-menstrual syndrome.' *Journal of Reproductive Medicine*, vol 32, no 6, pp. 435–41 (1987).

13 Gallant, M.P. et al. 'Pyridoxine and magnesium status in women with pre-menstrual syndrome.' *Nutrition Research*, vol 7, pp. 243–52 (1987).

14 Abraham, G.E. and Lubran, M.M. 'Serum and red cell magnesium levels in patients with pre-menstrual tension.' *American Journal of Clinical Nutrition*, vol 34, pp. 2364–6 (1981).

15 Rosenstein, D.L. et al. 'Magnesium measures across the menstrual cycle in pre-menstrual syndrome.' *Biological Psychiatry*, vol 35, pp. 557–61 (1994).

16 Schmidt, P.J. et al. 'Differential behavioural effects of gonadal steroids in women with and in those without pre-menstrual syndrome.' *New England Journal of Medicine*, vol 338, no 4, pp. 209–16 (1998).

Chapter 3: Diagnosing PMS

1 Kraemer, G.R. and Kraemer, R.R. 'Pre-menstrual syndrome: diagnosis and treatment experiences.' *Journal of Women's Health*, vol 7, no 7, pp. 893–907 (1998).

2 Rubinow, D.R. et al. 'Changes in plasma hormones across the menstrual cycle in patients with menstrually related mood disorders and in control subjects.' *American Journal of Obstetrics and Gynaecology*, vol 158, no 5–11 (1988).

3 Schmidt, P.J. et al. 'Lack of effect of induced menses on symptoms in women with pre-menstrual syndrome.' *New England Journal of Medicine*, vol 324, pp. 1174–9 (1991).

Chapter 4: The Conventional Approach to PMS

1 Trott, A. et al. 'Pre-menstrual syndrome: diagnosis and treatment.' *Delaware Medical Journal*, vol 68, no 7, pp. 357–63 (1996).

2 Bancroft, J. and Rennie, D. 'The impact of oral contraceptives on the experience of perimenstrual mood clumsiness, food craving and other symptoms.' *Journal of Psychosomatic Research*, vol 37, pp. 195–202 (1993).

3 Thomas, S. and Ellerton, C. 'Nuisance or natural and healthy: should monthly menstruation be optional for women?' *Lancet*, vol 355, pp. 9222–4 (2000).

4 West, C.P. and Hillier, H. 'Ovarian suppression with the gonadotrophin-releasing hormone agonist goserelin (Zoladex) in management of the pre-menstrual tension syndrome.' *Human Reproduction*, vol 9, pp. 1058–63 (1994).

5 Mortola, J.F. 'Applications of gonadotrophin-releasing hormone analogues in the treatment of pre-menstrual syndrome.' *Clinical Obstetrics and Gynaecology*, vol 36, pp. 753–63 (1993).

6 Carlton, G.J. and Burnett, J.W. 'Danazol and migraine.' *New England Journal of Medicine*, vol 310, p. 721 (1984).

7 O'Brien, P.M. and Abukhalil, I.E. 'Randomised controlled trial of the management of pre-menstrual syndrome and pre-menstrual mastalgia using luteal phase-only danazol.' *American Journal of Obstetrics and Gynaecology*, vol 180, pp. 18–23 (1999).

8 Watts, J.F. et al. 'A clinical trial using danazol for the treatment of pre-menstrual tension.' *British Journal of Obstetrics and Gynaecology*, vol 94, pp. 30–4 (1987).

9 Mira, M. et al. 'Mefenamic acid in the treatment of pre-menstrual syndrome.' *Obstetrics and Gynaecology*, vol 68, pp. 395–8 (1986) and Jakubowicz, D.L. et al. 'The treatment of pre-menstrual tension with mefenamic acid analysis of prostaglandin concentration.' *British Journal of Obstetrics and Gynaecology*, vol 91, pp. 79–84 (1984).

10 Wang, M. et al. 'Treatment of pre-menstrual syndrome by spironolactone: a double-blind, placebo-controlled study.' *Acta Obstetricia et Gynaecologica Scandinavica*, vol 74, pp. 803–8 (1995).

11 Magos, A.L. et al. 'Treatment of the pre-menstrual syndrome by subcutaneous oestradiol implants and cycle oral noresthisterone: placebo controlled study.' *British Medical Journal*, vol 292, pp. 1629–33 (1986).

12 Magos, A.L. et al. 'The effects of noresthisterone in post-menopausal women on oestrogen replacement therapy: A model for the pre-menstrual syndrome.' *British Journal of Obstetrics and Gynaecology*, vol 93, pp. 1290–6 (1986).

13 Bancroft, J. 'The pre-menstrual syndrome – a reappraisal of the concept and the evidence.' *Psychological Medicine*, monograph supplement 24, pp. 1–47 (1993).

14 Watson, N.R. et al. 'The long-term effects of oestradiol implant therapy for the treatment of pre-menstrual syndrome.' *Gynaecological Endocrinology*, vol 4, no 2, pp. 99–107 (1990).

15 Smith, R.N. et al. 'A randomised comparison over 8 months of 100mcg and 200mcg twice weekly doses of transdermal oestradiol in the treatment of severe pre-menstrual syndrome.' *British Journal of Obstetrics and Gynaecology*, vol 102, pp. 475–84 (1995).

16 Schairer, C. 'Menopausal oestrogen and oestrogen-progestogen replacement therapy and breast cancer risk.' *Journal of the American Medical Association*, vol 283, no 4, pp. 485–91 (2000).

17 Hammarback, S. et al. 'Relationship between symptom severity and hormone changes in women with pre-menstrual syndrome.' *Journal of Clinical Endocrinology and Metabolism*, vol 68, pp. 125–30 (1989).

18 Bancroft, J. and Backstrom, T. 'Pre-menstrual syndrome.' *Clinical Endocrinology*, vol 22, pp. 313–36 (1985).

19 Magill, P.J. 'Investigation of the efficacy of progesterone pessaries in the relief of symptoms of pre-menstrual syndrome.' Progesterone Study Group. *British Journal of General Practice*, vol 45, no 400, pp. 589–93 (1995).

20 Freeman, E. et al. 'Ineffectiveness of progesterone suppository treatment for pre-menstrual syndrome.' *Journal of the American Medical Association*, vol 264, pp. 349–53 (1990).

21 Grimes, D. 'Progestins, breast cancer and the limitations of epidemiology.' *Fertility and Sterility*, vol 57, no 3, pp. 492–3 (1992).

22 *International Journal of Cancer*, vol 92, pp. 469–73 (2001).

23 Grio, R. 'Clinical efficacy of tamoxifen in the treatment of pre-menstrual mastodynia' (translated from the Italian. *Minerva Ginecologica*, vol 50, no 3, pp. 101–3 (1998).

24 Harrison, W.M. et al. 'Treatment of pre-menstrual dysphoria with alprazolam: A controlled study.' *Archives of General Psychiatry*, vol 47, p. 270 (1990).

25 Dimmock, P. et al. 'Efficacy of selective serotonin-reuptake inhibitors in pre-menstrual syndrome: a systematic review.' *The Lancet*, vol 356, pp. 1131–6 (2000).

26. Magos, A.L. et al. 'Treatment of the pre-menstrual syndrome by subcutaneous oestradiol implants.' *British Medical Journal Clinical Research Edition*, 292, 6536, pp. 1629–33 (1986).

Part Two: The Natural Approach to Treating PMS
Chapter 5: The PMS Diet

1 Woods, N.F. et al. 'Major life events, daily stressors and perimenstrual symptoms.' *Nursing Research*, vol 34, pp. 263–7 (1985).

2 Nock, B. 'Norandrogenic regulation of progestin receptors: new findings, new questions, reproduction: a behavioural and neuroendocrine prospective.' *The Annals of the New York Academy of Sciences*, vol 474, no 415, p. 22 (1986).

3 Goei, G.S. 'Dietary patterns of patients with pre-menstrual tension.' *Journal of Applied Nutrition*, vol 34, pp. 4–11 (1982).

4 Wurtman, J.J. et al. 'Effect of nutrient intake on pre-menstrual depression.' *American Journal of Obstetrics and Gynaecology*, vol 161, no 5, pp. 1228–34 (1989).

5 Rossignol, A.M. and Bonnlander, H. 'Prevalence and severity of the pre-menstrual syndrome: Effects of foods and beverages that are sweet or high in sugar content.' *Journal of Reproductive Medicine*, vol 36, no 2, pp. 131–6 (1991).

6 Budd, M. *Low Blood Sugar.* Thorsons, London (1995).

7 Ringsdorf, W. et al. 'Sucrose, neutrophil phagocytosis and resistance to disease.' *Dental Survey*, vol 52, pp. 46–8 (1976).

8 Wurtman, R.J. 'Neurochemical changes following high dose aspartame with dietary carbohydrates.' *New England Journal of Medicine*, pp. 429–30 (1983).

9 Blundell, J.E. and Hill, A.J. 'Paradoxical effects of an intense sweetener (aspartame) on appetite.' *Lancet*, vol 1, 8489, pp. 1092–3 (1986).

10 Stegink, L.D. et al. 'Effect of repeated ingestion of aspartame-sweetened beverages on plasma amino acid, blood methanol and blood formate concentrations.' *Metabolism*, vol 38, no 4, pp. 357–63 (1989).

11 Lipton, S.A. and Rosenberg, P.A. 'Excitatory amino acids as a final common pathway for neurologic disorders.' *New England Journal of Medicine*, vol 300, no 9, pp. 613–22 (1994).

12 Minton, J.P. et al. 'Clinical and biochemical studies of methylxanthine-related fibrocystic breast disease.' *Surgery*, vol 90, pp. 299–304 (1981).

13 Horrobin, D.F. et al. 'Abnormalities in plasma essential fatty acid levels in women with pre-menstrual syndrome and with nonmalignant breast disease.' *Journal of Nutritional Medicine*, vol 2, pp. 259–64 (1991).

14 Mann, F.V. 'Metabolic consequences of dietary trans fatty acids.' *Lancet*, vol 343, no 8908, pp. 1268–71 (1994).

15 *American Journal of Clinical Nutrition*, vol 71, pp. 103–8 (2000).

16 Makela, S.I. et al. 'Dietary soybean may be antiestrogenic in mice.' *Journal of Nutrition,* vol 125, no 3 pp. 437–45 (1995).

17 Aldercreutz et al. 'Dietary phytoestrogens and cancer: in vitro and in vivo studies.' *Journal of Steroid Chemistry and Molecular Biology,* vol 3–8, no 41, pp. 331–7 (1992)

18 Barnard, N.D. et al. 'Diet and sex-hormone binding globulin, dysmenorrhea, and premenstrual syndrome.' *Obstetrics and Gynaecology,* vol 95, no 2, pp. 245–50 (2000).

19 Cassidy, A. et al. 'Biological effects of a diet of soy protein rich in isoflavones on the menstrual cycle of premenopausal women.' *American Journal of Clinical Nutrition,* vol 60, pp. 333–40 (1994).

20 Coleman, M.P. et al. *Trends in Cancer Incidence and Mortality.* IARC Publication no 121, Lyon, France (1993).

21 Anderson, J. et al. 'Meta-analysis of the effects of soy protein intake on serum lipids.' *New England Journal of Medicine,* vol 333, no 5, pp. 276–82 (1995).

22 Phipps, W.R. et al. 'Effect of flaxseed ingestion on the menstrual cycle.' *Journal of Clinical Endocrinology and Metabolism,* vol 77, no 5, pp. 1215–19 (1993).

Chapter 6: Lifestyle Changes

1 Boyce, N. 'Growing up too soon.' *New Scientist,* 2 August 1997, p. 5.

2 Campbell, J.M. and Harrison, K.L. 'Smoking and infertility' *Medical Journal of Australia,* vol 1, 8, pp. 342–3 (1979).

3 Jick, H. et al. 'Relation between smoking and age of natural menopause.' *Lancet,* vol 1, pp. 1354–5 (1977).

4 Hikon, H. et al. 'Antihepatoxic actions of flavonolignans from *Silybum marianum* fruits.' *Planta Medica,* vol 50, pp. 248–50 (1984).

5 Woods, N.F. et al. 'Major life events, daily stressors and perimenstrual symptoms.' *Nursing Research,* vol 34, pp. 263–7 (1985).

6 Barnea, E.R. and Tal, J. 'Stress-related reproductive failure.' *Journal of In Vitro Fertilisation and Embryo Transfer,* vol 8, pp. 15–23 (1991).

7 Franklin, M. et al. 'Neuroendocrine evidence for dopaminergic actions of Hypericum extract (LI160) in healthy volunteers.' *Biological Psychiatry,* vol 46, no 4, pp. 581–4 (1999).

8 Kuczmierczyk et al. 'Coping styles in women with pre-menstrual syndrome.' *Acta Psychiatrica Scandinavica,* vol 89, pp. 301–5 (1994).

9 Brown, J. 'Staying fit and staying well: Physical fitness as a moderator of life stress.' *Journal of Personality and Social Psychology,* vol 60, no 4, pp. 555–61 (1991).

10 Wolf, S. and Bruhn, J. *The Power of the Clan: The Influence of Human Relationshps on Heart Disease.* Transaction Publishers, Piscataway, New Jersey (1993).

11 Goodale, I.L. et al. 'Alleviation of pre-menstrual syndrome symptoms with the relaxation response.' *Obstetrics and Gynaecology,* vol 75, pp. 649–55 (1990).

12 Groer, M. and Ohnesorge, C. 'Menstrual cycle lengthening and reduction in premenstrual distress through guided imagery.' *Journal of Holistic Nursing,* vol 11, pp. 286–94 (1993).

13 Ben-Manachem, M. 'Treatment of dysmenorrhoea: A relaxation therapy program.' *International Journal of Gynaecology and Obstetrics,* vol 17, pp. 340–2 (1980).

14 Hernandez-Reif, M. et al. 'Pre-menstrual symptoms are relieved by massage therapy.' *Journal of Psychosomatic Obstetrics and Gynaecology,* vol 1, pp. 9–15 (2000).

15   Touch Research Institute of the University of Miami School of Medicine.

16 Spiegel, K. et al. 'Impact of sleep debt on metabolic and endocrine function.' *Lancet,* vol 354, pp. 1435–9 (1999).

17 Kahn, S.E. et al. 'Aetiology and pathogenesis of Type II diabetes mellitus and related disorders.' In Becker, K. (ed.) *Principles and Practice of Endocrinology and Metabolism*, pp. 1210–16. J.B. Lippincott (1995).

18 Kern, W. et al. 'Changes in cortisol and growth hormone secretion during nocturnal sleep in the course of ageing.' *Journal of Gerontology*, vol 51A, no M3–9 (1996).

19 Wyatt, R. 'Effects of L-tryptophan (a natural sedative) on human sleep.' *Lancet*, vol 2, pp. 842–6 (1970).

20 Johnson, W.G. et al. 'Macronutrient intake, eating habit and exercise as moderators of menstrual distress in healthy women.' *Psychosomatic Medicine*, vol 57, pp. 324–30 (1995).

21 Byrne, A. and Byrne, D.G. 'The effect of exercise on depression, anxiety and other mood states: a review.' *Journal of Psychosomatic Research*, vol 37, pp. 565–74 (1993).

22 Rapkin, A. and Laughlin, D. 'Guidelines for the diagnosis and treatment of pre-menstrual syndrome.' *Family Practice Recertification*, vol 21, no 1, pp. 42–70 (1999).

23 Steege, J.F. and Blumenthal, J.A. 'The effects of aerobic exercise on pre-menstrual symptoms in middle-aged women: A preliminary study.' *Journal of Psychosomatic Research*, vol 37, no 2, pp. 127–33 (1993).

24 Babyak, M. et al. 'Exercise maintenance of therapeutic benefits after 10 months'. *Psychosomatic Medicine*, vol 62, no 5, pp. 633–8 (2000).

25 Bernstein, L. et al. 'Physical exercise and reduced risk of breast cancer in young women.' *Journal of the National Cancer Institute*, vol 86, no 5, pp. 633–8 (1997).

Chapter 7: Food Supplements

1 Schroeder, H.A. 'Losses of vitamins and trace minerals, resulting from processing and preservation of foods.' *American Journal of Clinical Nutrition*, vol 24, pp. 562–73 (1971).

2 Tonkin, R.D. 'Role of Research in complementary medicine and therapy.' *Journal of Social Medicine*, vol 80, no 6, pp. 361–3 (1987).

3 Adams, P. et al. 'The effect of pyridoxine hydrochloride (vitamin B6) upon depression associated with oral contraception.' *Lancet*, vol 1, pp. 897–904 (1973).

4 Wyatt, K.M. 'Efficacy of vitamin B6 in the treatment of pre-menstrual syndrome: Systematic review.' *British Medical Journal*, vol 318, pp. 1375–81 (1999).

5 London, R.S. et al. 'Efficacy of alpha-tocopherol in the treatment of pre-menstrual syndrome.' *Journal of Reproductive Medicine*, vol 32, pp. 400–4 (1987).

6 Choung, C.J. 'Vitamin E levels in pre-menstrual syndrome.' *American Journal of Obstetrics and Gynaecology*, vol 164, pp. 1591–5 (1990).

7 Abraham, G.E. and Lubran, M.M. 'Serum and red cell magnesium levels in patients with pre-menstrual tension.' *American Journal of Clinical Nutrition*, vol 34, pp. 2364–6 (1981).

8 De Souza, M.C. et al. 'A synergistic effect of a daily supplement for one month of 200mg magnesium and 50mg vitamin B6 for the relief of anxiety-related pre-menstrual syndrome: A randomised double-blind, crossover study.' *Journal of Women's Health and Gender-Based Medicine*, vol 9, no 2, pp. 131–9 (2000).

9 Walker, A.F. et al. 'Magnesium supplementation alleviates pre-menstrual symptoms of fluid retention.' *Journal of Women's Health*, vol 7, no 9, pp. 1157–65 (1998).

10 Faccinetti, F. et al. 'Magnesium prophylaxis of menstrual migraine: effects on intracellular magnesium.' *Headache*, vol 31, pp. 298–304 (1991).

11 Mira, M. et al. 'Vitamin and trace element status in pre-menstrual syndrome.' *American Journal of Clinical Nutrition*, vol 47, pp. 636–41 (1988).

12 Rosenstein, D.L. et al. 'Magnesium measures across the menstrual cycle in pre-menstrual syndrome.' *Bio Psychiatry*, vol 35, pp. 557–61 (1994).

13 Thys-Jacobs, S. 'Calcium carbonate and the pre-menstrual syndrome: effects on pre-menstrual and menstrual symptoms.' Pre-menstrual Syndrome Study Group, *American Journal of Obstetrics and Gynaecology*, vol 179, no 2, pp. 444–52 (1998).

14 Thys-Jacobs, S. 'Micronutrients and the pre-menstrual syndrome: the case of calcium.' *Journal of the American College of Nutrition*, vol 19, no 2, pp. 220–7 (2000).

15 Thys-Jacobs, S. 'Vitamin D and calcium in menstrual migraine.' *Headache*, vol 34, no 9, pp. 544–6 (1994).

16 Chuong, C.J. and Dawson, E.B. 'Zinc and copper levels in pre-menstrual syndrome.' *Fertility and Sterility*, vol 62, pp. 313–20 (1994).

17 Balch, J. and Balch, P. *Prescription for Nutritional Healing*, G.P. Putnam and Sons, USA (1998).

18 Evans, G.W. and Pouchnik, D.J. 'Composition and biological activity of chromium-pyridine carboxylate complexes.' *Journal of Inorganic Biochemistry*, vol 49, pp. 177–87 (1993).

19 Anderson, R.A. 'Chromium, glucose tolerance and diabetes.' *Biological Trace Element Research*, vol 32, pp. 19–24 (1992).

20 Anderson, R.A. et al. 'Effects of supplemental chromium on patients with symptoms of reactive hypoglycaemia.' *Metabolism*, vol 36, pp. 351–5 (1987).

21 Horrobin, D.F. et al. 'Abnormalities in plasma essential fatty acid levels in women with pre-menstrual syndrome and with nonmalignant breast disease.' *Journal of Nutritional Medicine*, vol 2, pp. 259–64 (1991).

22 Puolakka, J. et al. 'Biochemical and clinical effects of treating the pre-menstrual syndrome with prostaglandin synthesis precursors.' *Journal of Reproductive Medicine*, vol 30, pp. 149–53 (1985).

23 Graham, J. *Evening Primrose Oil*, pp. 37–8. Thorsons, London (1984).

24 McFayden, I.J. et al. 'Cyclical breast pain – some observations and the difficulties in treatment.' *British Journal of Clinical Practice*, vol 46, pp. 161–4 (1992).

25 Clare, A. 'Pre-menstrual syndrome: single or multiple causes?' *Canadian Journal of Psychiatry*, vol 30, pp. 474–82 (1985).

26 Magnussen, I.E. and Nielsen-Kudsk, F. 'Bioavailability and related pharmacokinetics in man of orally administered L-5-hydroxytryptophan in a steady state.' *Acta Pharmacologica et Toxicologica*, vol 46, pp. 257–62 (1980).

27 Poldinger, B. et al. 'A functional-dimensional approach to depression: Serotonin deficiency as a target syndrome in a comparison of 5-hydroxytryptophan and fluvoxamine.' *Psychopathology*, vol 24, pp. 53–81 (1991).

Chapter 8: Herbs

1 Schellenberg, R. 'Treatment for the pre-menstrual syndrome with agnus fruit extract: prospective, randomised, placebo controlled study.' *British Medical Journal*, vol 322, pp. 134–7 (2001).

2 Sliutz, G. et al. 'Agnus castus extracts inhibit prolactin secretion of rat pituitary cells.' *Hormone and Metabolic Research*, vol 25, pp. 253–5 (1993).

3 Sheu, S.J. et al. 'Analysis and processing of Chinese herbal drugs IV: The study of *Angelicae radix*.' *Planta Medica*, vol 53, pp. 377–8 (1987).

4 Qi-bing, M. et al. 'Advance in the pharmacological studies of radix Angelica sinensis (oliv) diels (Chinese danggui).' *Chinese Medicine Journal*, vol 104, pp. 776–81 (1991).

5 Zhu, D.P.Q. 'Dong quai.' *American Journal of Chinese Medicine*, vol 15, pp. 117–25 (1987).

6 Hikon, H. et al. 'Antihepatoxic actions of flavonolignans from *Silybum marianum* fruits.' *Planta Medica*, vol 50, pp. 248–50 (1984).

7 Bosisio, E. et al. 'Effect of the flavonolignans of *Silybum marianum* L on lipid peroxidation in rat liver microsomes and freshly isolated hepatocytes.' *Pharmacology Research*, vol 25, no 2, pp. 147–54 (1992).

8 Hruby, K. et al. 'Chemotherapy of *Amanita phalloides* poisoning with intravenous silibinin.' *Human Toxicology*, vol 2, pp. 183–95 (1983).

9 Linde, E. et al. 'St John's wort for depression – an overview and meta-analysis of randomised clinical trials.' *British Medical Journal*, vol 313, pp. 253–61 (1996).

10 Stevinson, C. and Ernst, E. 'A pilot study of *Hypericum perforatum* for the treatment of pre-menstrual syndrome.' *British Journal of Obstetrics and Gynaecology*, vol 107, no 7, pp. 870–6 (2000).

11 Woelk, H. 'Comparison of St John's wort and imipramine for treating depression: randomised controlled trial.' *British Medical Journal*, vol 321, pp. 536–9 (2000).

12 Sergio, W. 'A natural food, malabar tamarind, may be effective in the treatment of obesity.' *Medical Hypotheses*, vol 27, p. 40 (1988).

Chapter 9: The Treatment Alternatives

1 Parry, B.L. et al. 'Light therapy of late luteal phase dysphoric disorder: An extended study.' *American Journal of Psychiatry*, vol 150, no 9, pp. 1417–19 (1993).

2 Kroger, W.S. and Schneider, A.S. 'An electronic aid for hypnotic induction: A preliminary report.' *Journal of Clinical and Experimental Hypnosis*, vol 7, pp. 93–8 (1959).

3 Walter, V.J. and Walter, W.G. 'The central effects of rhythmic sensory stimulation.' *Electro-encephalography and Clinical Neurophysiology*, vol 1, pp. 57–86 (1949).

4 Anderson, D.J. et al. 'Preliminary trial of photic stimulation for pre-menstrual syndrome.' *Journal of Obstetrics and Gynaecology*, vol 17, no 1, pp. 76–9 (1997).

5 Folkard, S. et al. 'Can melatonin improve shift workers' tolerance of the night shift? Some preliminary findings.' *Chronobiology International*, vol 10, no 5, pp. 315–20 (1993).

6 Blake, F. et al. 'Cognitive therapy for pre-menstrual syndrome: a controlled trial.' *Journal of Psychosomatic Research*, vol 45, no 4, pp. 307–18 (1998).

7 Chapman, E.H. et al. 'Results of the homeopathic treatment of PMS.' *Journal of the American Institute of Homeopaths*, vol 87, no 1, p. 14, 21 (1994).

8 Oleson, T. and Flocco, W. 'Randomised controlled study of pre-menstrual symptoms treated with ear, hand and foot reflexology.' *Obstetrics and Gynaecology*, vol 82, pp. 906–11 (1993).

9 Cutler, W.B. et al. 'Human axillary secretions influence women's menstrual cycles: The role of donor extract from men.' *Hormones and Behavior*, vol 20, pp. 463–73 (1986).

Chapter 10: Coping with the Symptoms

1 Schinfeld, J.S. 'PMS and candidiasis: Study explores possible link.' *Female Patient*, July 1987, p. 66.

2 Faccinetti, F. et al. 'Magnesium prophylaxis of menstrual migraine: Effects on intracellular magnesium.' *Headache*, vol 31, pp. 298–304 (1991).

3 Glucek, C.J. et al. 'Amelioration of severe migraine with Omega 3 fatty acids: A double-blind, placebo controlled clinical trial.' *American Journal of Clinical Nutrition*, vol 43, p. 710 (1986).

4 Johnson, E.S. et al. 'Efficacy of feverfew as prophylactic treatment of migraine.' *British Medical Journal*, vol 291, pp. 569–73 (1985).

5 Vaughn, T.R. 'The role of food in the pathogenesis of migraine headache.' *Clinical Reviews in Allergy*, vol 12, pp. 167–80 (1994).

6 Janiger, O. et al. 'Cross cultural study of pre-menstrual symptoms.' *Psychosomatics*, vol 13, pp. 226–35 (1972).

7 Minton, J.P. et al. 'Clinical and biochemical studies of methylxanthine-related fibrocystic breast disease.' *Surgery*, vol 90, pp. 299–304 (1981).

8 Petrakis, N.L. and King, E.B. 'Cytological abnormalities in nipple aspirates of breast fluid from women with severe constipation.' *Lancet*, vol 2, no 8257, pp. 1203–4 (1981).

9 London, R. et al. 'Mammary dysplasia: Endocrine parameters and tocopherol therapy.' *Nutrition Research*, vol 7, p. 243 (1982).

10 Pye, J.K. et al. 'Clinical experience of drug treatments for mastalgia.' *Lancet*, vol 2, pp. 373–7 (1985).

11 McFayden, I.J. et al. 'Cyclical breast pain – some observations and the difficulties in treatment.' *British Journal of Clinical Practice*, vol 46, pp. 161–4 (1992).

12 Kaizer, L. et al. 'Fish consumption and breast cancer risk.' *Nutrition And Cancer*, vol 12, pp. 61–68 (1989) and Cave, W.T. 'Dietary omega-3 polyunsaturated fats and breast cancer.' *Nutrition*, vol 12, no 1, pp. S39–S42 (1996).

13 Tamborini, A. and Taurelle, R. 'Value of standardised *Ginkgo biloba* extract (EGB 761) in the management of congestive symptoms of pre-menstrual syndrome.' *Revue Francaise de Gynécologie et d'Obstétrique*, vol 88, no 7–9, pp. 447–57 (1993).

14 Dalton, K. 'Menstruation and accidents.' *British Medical Journal*, vol 2, pp. 1425–6 (1960).

15 Kleijnen, J. and Knipschild, P. 'Ginkgo biloba.' *Lancet*, vol 340, pp. 1136–9 (1992).

16 Slayden, S.M. et al. 'Hyperandrogenemia in patients presenting with acne.' *Fertility and Sterility*, vol 75, no 5, pp. 889–92 (2001).

17 Aldercreutz, H. et al. 'Dietary phytoestrogens and cancer: in vitro and in vivo studies.' *Journal of Steroid Chemistry and Molecular Biology*, vol 3–8, no 41, pp. 331–7 (1992).

18 DiSilverio, F. et al. 'Evidence that *Serenoa repens* extract displays antiestrogenic activity in prostatic tissue of benign prostatic hypertrophy.' *European Urology*, vol 21, pp. 309–14 (1992).

19 Snider, B. and Dieteman, D. 'Pyridoxine therapy for pre-menstrual acne flare.' *Archives of Dermatology*, vol 110, pp. 130–1 (1974).

20 Chuong, C.J. and Dawson, E.B. 'Zinc and copper levels in pre-menstrual syndrome.' *Fertility and Sterility*, vol 62, pp. 313–20 (1994).

Chapter 11: Could There Be Another Cause?

1 Schinfeld, J.S. 'PMS and candidiasis: Study explores possible link.' *Female Patient*, July 1987, p. 66.

2 Hilton, E. et al. 'Ingestion of yoghurt containing lactobacillus acidophilus as prophylaxis for candidal vaginitis.' *Annals of Internal Medicine*, vol 116, no 5, pp. 353–7 (1992).

3 Mikhail, M.S. et al. 'Decreased beta-carotene levels in exfoliated vaginal epithelia cells in women with vaginal candidiasis.' *American Journal of Reproductive Immunology*, vol 32, pp. 221–5 (1994).

4 Edman, J. et al. 'Zinc status in women with recurrent vulvovaginal candidiasis.' *American Journal of Obstetrics and Gynaecology*, vol 155, no 5, pp. 1082–5 (1986).

5 Das, U.N. 'Antibiotic-like action of essential fatty acids.' *Canadian Medical Association Journal*, vol 132, no 12, p. 1350 (1985).

6 Adetumbi, M. et al. '*Allium sativum* (garlic) inhibits lipid synthesis by candida albicans.' *Antimicrobial Agents and Chemotherapy*, vol 30, no 3, pp. 499–501 (1986).

7 Amin, A. et al. 'Berberine sulfate: antimicrobial activity, bioassay and mode of action.' *Canadian Journal of Microbiology*, vol 15, pp. 1067–76 (1969).

8   Pena, E. '*Melaleuca alternifolia* oil: its use for trichomonal vaginitis and other vaginal infections.' *Obstetrics and Gynaecology*, vol 19, no 6, pp. 793–5 (1962).

9   Coeuginet, E. and Kuhnast, R. 'Recurrent candidiasis: Adjuvant immunotherapy with different formulations of Echinacin (R).' *Therapiewoche*, vol 36, pp. 3352–8 (1986).

10 Brayshaw, N.D. and Brayshaw, D.D. 'Thyroid hypofunction in pre-menstrual syndrome.' *New England Journal of Medicine*, vol 315, pp. 1486–7 (1986).

11 Schmidt et al. 'Thyroid function in women with pre-menstrual syndrome.' *Journal of Clinical Endocrinology and Metabolism*, vol 76, pp. 671–4 (1993).

12 Brayshaw, N.D. and Brayshaw, D.D. 'Thyroid hypofunction.'

13 Yamamoto, I. et al. 'Anti-tumour effects of seaweed.' *Japanese Journal of Experimental Medicine*, vol 44, pp. 543–6 (1974).

14 Iritani, N. and Nagi, S. 'Effects of spinach and wakeame on cholesterol turnover in the rat.' *Atherosczerosis*, vol 15, pp. 87–92 (1972).

15 Olivieri, O. et al. 'Low selenium status in the elderly influences thyroid hormones.' *Clinical Science*, vol 89, pp. 637–42 (1995).

Chapter 12: Tests

1   Schinfeld, J.S. 'PMS and candidiasis: Study explores possible link.' *Female Patient*, July 1987, p. 66.

2   Suzuki, T. and Yamamoto, P. 'Organic mercury levels in human hair with and without storage for eleven years.' *Bulletin of Environmental Contamination and Toxicology*, vol 28, pp. 186–8 (1982).

3   James, V. 'Using hair to screen for breast cancer.' *Nature*, vol 398, no 6722, pp. 33–4 (1999).

4   Dickman, M.D. and Leung, K.M. 'Mercury and organochlorine exposure from fish consumption in Hong Kong.' *Chemosphere*, vol 37, no 5, pp. 991–1015 (1998).

Staying in Touch

If you have any health problems and are interested in finding a more natural approach to treating them, or would like to find out what supplements and tests are available to you, please feel free to contact me and I will send you more information on how you can help yourself.

Workshops, cassettes and videos

I give workshops and talks around the world and have produced cassettes and videos from some of these. Please call if you would like to find out more about future workshops and/or recordings and you will be sent an information pack.

Consultations

If you want to see or talk to someone personally, I am available for private consultations at the following clinics: The Hale Clinic, Regent's Park, London and at Women's Healthcare, St John's Wood, London and postal consultations can be arranged.

For appointments and enquiries contact me at:
Dr Marilyn Glenville, Nevill Estate, Danegate, Eridge Green, Tunbridge Wells, Kent, TN3 9JA.
Tel: 01892 750511 Fax: 01892 750533
website: www.marilynglenville.com
email: health@marilynglenville.com

If you would like to hear more advice from Dr Glenville on any of the following subjects:

- **Natural alternatives to dieting** *How to lose weight naturally*
- **Natural alternatives to HRT** *How to stay healthy through the menopause and prevent osteoporosis*
- **Natural solutions to infertility** *How to increase your chances of conceiving and preventing miscarriages*

then call **0906 7010030** and choose the information you would like to hear.

Calls are charged at 50p per minute at all times.
Helpline No: 01892 750511.

Suggested Reading

The 30 Day Fat Burner Diet, Patrick Holford (Piatkus, 1999)
Feminisation of Nature, Deborah Cadbury (Penguin Books, 1998)
How to Avoid GM Food, Joanna Blythman (Fourth Estate, 1999)
Low Blood Sugar, Martin Budd (Thorsons, 1997)
Natural Alternatives to Dieting, Marilyn Glenville (Kyle Cathie, 1999)
Natural Alternatives to HRT Cookbook, Marilyn Glenville (Kyle Cathie, 2000)
Nutritional Health Handbook for Women, Marilyn Glenville (Piatkus, 2001)
Our Stolen Future, Theo Colborn, Dianne Dumanoski and John Peterson (Abacus, 1997)
The PMS Bible, Katharina Dalton (Vermilion, 1999)
Silent Spring, Rachel Carson (Penguin Books, 1999 [reprint]

Useful Addresses

Acupuncture
The British Acupuncture Council
63 Jeddo Road
London W12 9HQ
Tel: 020 8735 0400
Fax: 020 8735 0404

Cognitive Behavioural Therapy (CBT)
Section of Psychopharmacology
Institute of Psychiatry
De Crespigny Park
London SE5 8AF

Homeopathy
Society of Homeopaths
4a Artizan Road
Northampton NN1 4HU
Tel: 01604 621400

Medical Herbalism
National Institute of Medical Herbalism
56 Longbrook Street
Exeter EX4 6AH
Tel: 01392 426022

Nutrition
British Association of Nutritional Therapists
27 Old Gloucester Street
London WC1N 3XX
Tel/Fax: 0870 6061284

Osteopathy
General Osteopathic Council
Osteopathy House
176 Tower Bridge Road
London SE1 3LU
Tel: 020 7357 6655

General
Nutri Centre
7 Park Crescent
London W1N 3HF
Tel: 020 7436 5122

Verity – The Polycystic Self-Help Group
Trindlemanor
52–54 Featherstone Street
London EC1Y 8RT

What Doctors Don't Tell You (monthly newsletter, sold by subscription)
Satellite House
2 Salisbury Road
London SW19 4EZ
For subscriptions, tel: 01858 438894

Women's Healthcare
St John's Wood
27A Queen's Terrace
London NW8 5EA
Tel: 020 7483 0099

Index

Note: page numbers in *italic* refer to diagrams, page numbers in **bold** refer to information presented in tables.